Bacillus subtilis - Functionalities and One Health Applications

Edited by Hary Razafindralambo

Published in London, United Kingdom

Bacillus subtilis - Functionalities and One Health Applications
http://dx.doi.org/10.5772/intechopen.110978
Edited by Hary Razafindralambo

Contributors
Ayten Yazgan-Karataş, Bushra Mustafa, Dilan Ergün, Göksu Tartar, Hary Razafindralambo, Holy Rabetafika, Humaira Mushtaq Mukadam, Hussnain Ahmed Janjua, Mehwish Malik, Mohamadsadegh Mohamadzadeh, Sajid Iqbal, Sakineh Abbaspour, Shikha Vikrant Gaikwad, Sonam Shrirang Shinde, Vijayaram Seerengaraj, Viraj Vivek Gaonkar

First published in London, United Kingdom, 2025 by IntechOpen
IntechOpen is the global imprint of INTECHOPEN LIMITED, registered in England and Wales, registration number: 11086078, 167-169 Great Portland Street, London, W1W 5PF, United Kingdom

For EU product safety concerns: IN TECH d.o.o., Prolaz Marije Krucifikse Kozulić 3, 51000 Rijeka, Croatia, info@intechopen.com or visit our website at intechopen.com.

British Library Cataloguing-in-Publication Data
A catalogue record for this book is available from the British Library

Bacillus subtilis - Functionalities and One Health Applications
Edited by Hary Razafindralambo
p. cm.
Print ISBN 978-1-83634-185-7
Online ISBN 978-1-83634-184-0
eBook (PDF) ISBN 978-1-83634-186-4

Meet the editor

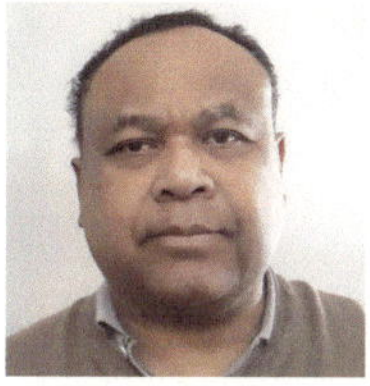

Hary L. Razafindralambo is currently head of e-Lab (ProBioLab) of multidisciplinary science and technology, and PI of international projects at the University of Liege - Gembloux Agro-Bio Tech in Belgium. He received a Ph.D. degree in Agronomic Sciences and Biological Engineering (1996) and graduated as a Chemist and Agroindustry engineer (1990) from Gembloux Agricultural University. His research and teaching expertise are the physical chemistry of biological and food systems, focusing on colloid and interface sciences, synergism, and interactions among functional biotic systems, including probiotics, prebiotics, postbiotics, and synbiotics. He supervises master's and Ph.D. students and postdoctoral international visitor researchers in this field. He recently assumed the role of editor for the book titled "Trends in Probiotic Applications" and the two Special Issues "Probiotics and their Metabolites" and "Role of Probiotics in Human Health" for Biomolecules, while being the founder of the journal "Current Probiotics".

Contents

Preface

Bacillus subtilis stands out as a beneficial and health-promoting microorganism with wide-ranging impacts on humans, animals, and plants, as well as their surrounding ecosystems, including soil, air, and water. Its versatile properties and functionalities render it a potential probiotic candidate for the One Health concept, which aims to reduce the risks of new emerging infectious diseases at the animal-human-ecosystem interface, antimicrobial resistance development, biodiversity loss, and the increase of synthetic agricultural inputs. Consequently, *B. subtilis* is crucial in shaping health, nutrition, ecology, and the economy worldwide.

This book deals with the most relevant and multiple basic properties, functionalities, and probiotic power of *Bacillus subtilis* and the myriad of bioactive extracellular metabolites it can produce within the context of One Health into three distinct sections.

Section 1 proposes a biochemical classification of the extracellular metabolites from *B. subtilis* and their functionalities that are relevant to One Health applications, while discussing the safety and regulation aspects (Chapter 1).

Section 2 focuses on the probiotic power of *Bacillus subtilis* by elucidating the mechanisms of action and offering insights into its health benefits for humans, animals, plants, applications and prospects (Chapter 2 and Chapter 3).

Section 3 examines the clinical and therapeutical, agricultural, and environmental potential applications of *Bacillus subtilis* by focusing on the antimicrobe, anticancer, and vaccine carrier (Chapter 4), as well as the biofertilizer, biocontrol, depolluting activities (Chapter 5) of its peptide and non-peptide active compounds.

The book addresses comprehensive, appropriate, and current information with basic and applied aspects intended for academic, undergraduate and graduate students, organizations, industrials, and practitioners.

Dr. Ing. Hary Razafindralambo Ph.D.
Gembloux Agro-Bio Tech,
University of Liege,
Gembloux, Belgium

Section 1

B. subtilis Extracellular Metabolites and Functionalities for One Health

Chapter 1

Bacillus subtilis: A Promising Bacterial Candidate for One Health Applications

Hary Razafindralambo, Vijayaram Seerengaraj and Holy Rabetafika

Abstract

Bacillus subtilis is widely recognized as a beneficial and safe microbe for both living species and the environment due to its broad spectrum of bioactive properties. Used for decades as a probiotic, *B. subtilis* produces diverse bioactive metabolites with antimicrobial, antitumor, antioxidant, and immunomodulatory activities. It forms resilient biofilms, sporulates under stress, promotes plant growth, enhances nutrient uptake, controls pathogens, and contributes to the bioremediation of environmental pollutants such as heavy metals and hydrocarbons. Its long-standing use in food fermentation supports its safety profile and recognition as a safe organism in various applications. Consequently, *B. subtilis* stands out as a promising candidate for achieving optimal "One Health" outcomes for humans, animals, plants, and their interconnected ecosystems. This chapter provides a biochemical classification of the metabolites and derivatives produced by *B. subtilis*, highlighting their properties and functions that offer health benefits to both living organisms and the environment.

Keywords: metabolites, probiotics, peptides, enzymes, antimicrobe, nutraceuticals, safety

1. Introduction

Faced with recent global disease outbreaks such as COVID-19, there has been a growing adoption of a One Health approach that considers how environmental changes influence the risks of infectious and chronic diseases for humans, animals, and plants. Therefore, designing adaptive, forward-looking, and multidisciplinary solutions to these challenges is necessary, with more preventive actions by addressing the root causes and drivers of infectious diseases, particularly at the animal-human-ecosystem interface. One Health approaches, such as reducing synthetic agricultural inputs and increasing biodiversity, present a global strategic framework to reduce the risks of new emerging infectious diseases at the animal-human-ecosystem interface. By focusing on preventive solutions, One Health contributes to better living species health and a more sustainable environment in the future [1].

The exploration of beneficial microbes appears to be an interesting route in One Health initiatives, bridging the realms of human, animal, plant, and environmental health throughout the world [2]. *B. subtilis*, a Gram-positive and spore-forming bacterium, is recognized among these beneficial microbes to the living species and their environment for its multiple properties and functions, as well as its broad versatility in various sectors such as medicine, agriculture, and environmental sciences [3]. This bacterial species acts in promoting health in direct and indirect manners by preventing and treating many diseases in humans and animals by producing and converting organic substrates into a wide range of bioactive metabolites, including antimicrobial peptides, enzymes, vitamins, exopolysaccharides, and volatile organic compounds [4]. It is also capable of forming complex and robust biofilms involved, for instance, in the protection of nerve cells and in long and healthy human longevity [5]. *B. subtilis* sporulates and survives in hostile conditions, high temperature, and acidic environment conditions, while being harmless to bacteria, making them effective food and feed ingredients [6, 7]. It also promotes plant growth and controls pathogens and pests responsible for plant diseases and damage [8], helps nutrient absorption from soil [9], and remediates the environment from toxic compounds [10]. One of its emerging and innovative applications is the capacity to synthesize nanoparticles [11], which have numerous applications [12]. Moreover, *B. subtilis* has been widely used as a cell factory for the industrial production of bioactive compounds, owing to a highly efficient protein secretion system and adaptable metabolism [13]. Consequently, *B. subtilis* has many assets to be a suitable bacterial candidate to reach optimal "One Health" for humans, animals, plants, and the related ecosystem.

This chapter overviews (1) the bioactive metabolites of *B. subtilis* and their roles in One Health, (2) the properties and applications of *B. subtilis* that are relevant to One Health, and finally (3) the safety and regulation aspects of its applications.

2. Metabolites of *B. subtilis* and their roles in One Health

B. subtilis has been well-known for the last decades as a producer of a variety of bioactive compounds, either primary metabolites, which are essential for proper bacterial growth, or secondary metabolites produced during the stationary phase of growth. Secondary metabolites are not essential for cell growth but provide competitive or adaptive advantages for both experimental and industrial uses [14]. *Bacillus subtilis* offers several technological advantages, such as a rapid growth rate, an ease of genetic manipulation, and a wealth of accumulated experimental data. It can serve as a tool for producing bioactive compounds for which the applications cover agriculture, medicine, biomaterials, and many industrial sectors such as cosmetics, food, textile, paint, and detergent, and can therefore provide benefits to humans, animals, plants, and the environment. It is not surprising that *B. subtilis* is appearing as a potential candidate for playing a pivotal role in One Health. Bioactive metabolites from *B. subtilis* can be classified according to several criteria, among others, their molecular structures, biosynthetic pathways, or based on their beneficial functionalities to the host. Chemical structure classification has its importance in terms of rational design through the structure-activity relationship investigations for searching for the most efficient biological activities or for increasing the knowledge on bioactive metabolite action mechanisms. According to their biosynthetic pathways, *B. subtilis* secondary metabolites can be categorized into non-ribosomal and ribosomal peptides, polyketides, and hybrid and volatile metabolites, which are further classified into different subclasses, as reviewed in detail in Ref. [15].

In this section, a classification based on the chemical structure, biochemical traits (proteins, carbohydrates, lipids, small organic and inorganic compounds, nanoparticles, and vesicles), and functionalities of the different categories of bioactive compounds is described. Some of the representative biomolecules for each class are illustrated in **Figure 1**.

2.1 Peptides and enzymes

Among the most important bioactive compounds from *B. subtilis* are those composed of amino acids linked by peptide bonds. These include cyclic and linear lipopeptides, peptides, and polypeptides, as well as lytic and quorum quenching enzymes and amino acids as monomers. Cyclic lipopeptides mainly belong to three families, surfactins, iturins, and fengycins, which contain 7–10 amino acid residues cyclized by β-hydroxy or β-amino fatty acid chains with a lactone or amide bond, respectively. These biomolecules exist in homologous series varying in fatty acid chain length (12–18 carbon atoms) and configuration (linear, iso, or anteiso) and in isoforms with various amino acid residues with L and D configurations [16]. For linear lipopeptides, we can find siderophores (e.g., bacillibactin) [17], gageopeptides from a marine *B. subtilis* strain [18], and subtilin, and other peptides such as dihyroisocoumarins, bacilysin, chlorotetain, and rhizocticins, which contain two or more amino acid residues, with or without other compounds in their structure. Polypeptides consist of polymers containing one amino acid residue, such as poly-γ-glutamic acid [19].

Enzymes secreted by *B. subtilis* can be categorized into lytic enzymes such as proteases, chitinases, glucanases, and amylases, and those involved in quorum quenching, that is, those that have the capacity to inactivate the production of signal or quorum sensing molecules (e.g., N-acyl-homoserine lactones) responsible for the growth of deleterious microbial pests. These enzymes are, for instance, lactonase, decarboxylase, acylase, and deaminase [4]. A particular lytic enzyme produced by

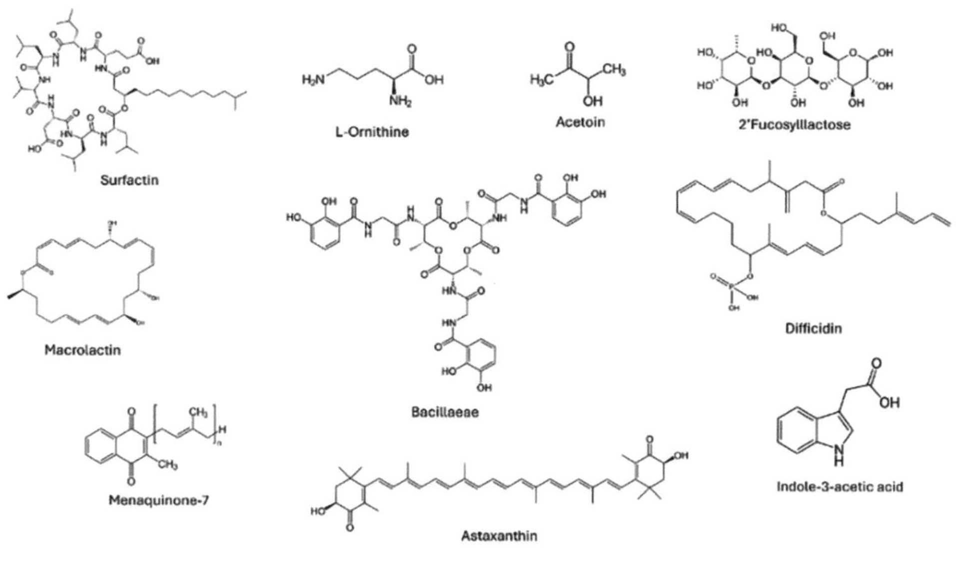

Figure 1.
Chemical structures of representative compounds for each category.

B. subtilis natto is nattokinase, which is a fibrinolytic serine protease found in Korean and Japanese foods [20].

Amino acid monomers such as L-Ornithine [21] and L-tryptophane [22] can be overproduced by *B. subtilis* strains for use in human health.

2.2 Polyketides

Polyketides (PKs) represent bioactive metabolites with diverse structures that contain an alternative methylene and carbonyl group [23]. This class of biomolecules has a multitude of activities encompassing antimicrobial, antitumor, and immunosuppressive effects [4]. Typical PKs produced by *B. subtilis* are difficidins and macrolactins, which are macrocyclic polyenes, and bacillaene, which is largely a linear compound. Difficidins are known for their broad-spectrum antibacterial activities, whereas macrolactins have activities against methicillin-resistant *Staphylococcus aureus* [24], and bacillaene can inhibit various fungi such as *Myxococcus xanthus* and *Trichoderma spp*. [25].

2.3 Carbohydrate-based compounds

B. subtilis produces carbohydrate-based metabolites such as exopolysaccharides (EPS) and oligosaccharides, which are substrate-dependent production. EPS are carbohydrate-based biopolymers with multiple structures and functions, which are excreted either in bound form around the cell surface (capsular EPSs) or in free form into the medium of cell growth (slime EPSs) [26]. *B. subtilis* has been reported to produce EPS (e.g., levan and hyaluronic acid) and prebiotic oligosaccharides such as fructooligosaccharides [27] and 2′-fucosyllactose [28]. This category of *B. subtilis* metabolites can exert anticancer, antioxidant, antibacterial, anti-inflammatory, and immunomodulatory activities [29].

2.4 Terpenes and terpenoid derivatives

B. subtilis is known for its ability to produce isoprene ($C5H8$ units), the simple form of a terpenoid molecule, and other important terpenoid compounds with particular importance for human and animal health, such as carotenoids, amorphadiene, taxadiene, and menaquinone-7 (MK-7), by means of engineered strains [30]. Terpenoids are mostly lipophilic compounds, considered volatile organic metabolites with a low boiling point and high vapor pressure, and exist in a diverse structural class of linear, cyclic, or polycyclic compounds, which generate multiple biological activities [31].

2.5 Small organic and inorganic compounds (<500 Da)

These bioactive metabolites produced by *B. subtilis* include volatile organic and inorganic compounds having a low molecular mass (< 500 Da). One of the most important categories is represented by organic acids, fatty acids, and derivatives, and other categories of small organic compounds [4]. The distribution of volatile secondary metabolites from *B. subtilis* has been reviewed [32]. The most abundant volatile secondary metabolites produced by *B. subtilis* can be classified according to their functional group as follows: ketones 15%, nitrogen-containing compounds 14%, hydrocarbons 14%, aromatic compounds 14%, and alcohols 11%.

Volatile inorganic compounds produced by *B. subtilis* are mainly gaseous by-products of primary metabolism, such as carbonated (CO2, CO), hydrogenated (H2), sulfur (H2S), or nitrogen (N2, NH3, NO)-containing compounds [4]. Particular attention is addressed to nitric oxide (NO) for its role in human longevity [33].

2.6 Nanoparticles

B. subtilis is also able to synthesize nanoparticles during incubation time after cultivation through metal ion reductases, such as iron oxide, for reducing arsenic toxicity in rice plants [11] and silver nanoparticles for depolluting water [34].

2.7 Extracellular vesicles

B. subtilis produces extracellular cell-derived membrane-surrounded vesicles (EVs) carrying bioactive molecules such as proteins and nucleic acids. Their average sizes range from 20 to 100 nm in diameter. EVs find applications as immunostimulants, adjuvants, or even vaccine vehicles, particularly in the aquaculture sector [35].

In terms of functionality, these metabolites can play essential roles in One Health approaches (**Figure 2**). They contribute to improved health outcomes across humans, animals, and plants, while also promoting a safer environment, either directly or indirectly. Their multiple activities and functionalities include antimicrobial, antioxidant, antitumor, immunostimulatory, and anti-inflammatory effects for preventing and treating various human infections and diseases. Additionally, they enhance nutrient availability, support plant growth and stress resistance, and aid in the degradation or immobilization of soil contaminants such as heavy metals and hydrocarbons.

Recognized as probiotics, *B. subtilis* finds many applications in food and feed as a supplement ingredient for promoting human and animal health, including both

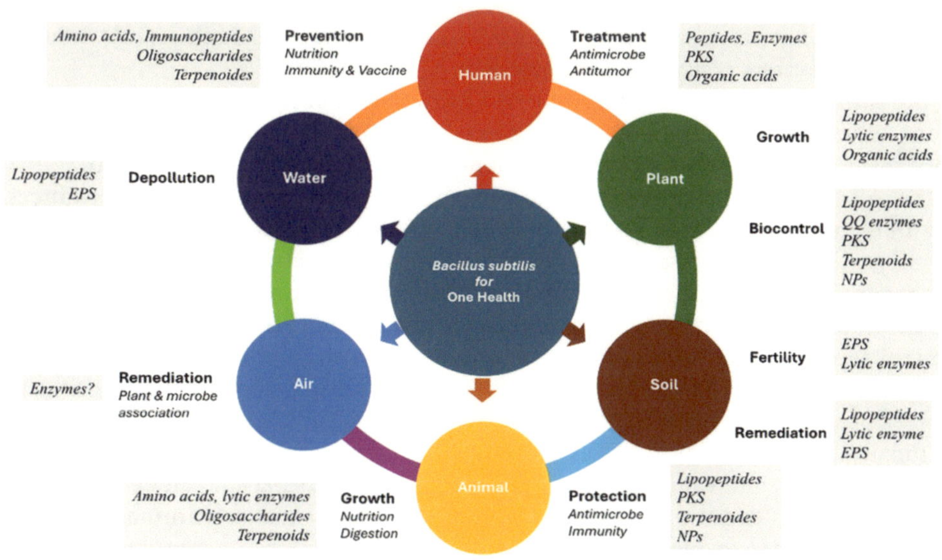

Figure 2.
B. subtilis *metabolites in One Health – EPS: Exopolysaccharides; QQ: quorum quenching; PKS: Polyketides; NPs: Nanoparticles.*

husbandry and aquatic animals [36]. Besides their use as experimental models and microbial cell factories by humans, the species *B. subtilis* var. natto is the main functional ingredient for fermented soybean foods such as Japanese natto [37], Korean cheonggukjang [35], and Chinese douche [38].

For humans and animals, most metabolites from *B. subtilis* can be used as nutraceuticals, providing both nutritional and pharmaceutical functions, and as therapeutic/antibiotic agents. Bioactive peptides such as cyclic lipopeptides (e.g., surfactin) are active against microbial infections (virus, bacteria, and fungi), especially against drug-resistant pathogens and cancer cells, inducing apoptosis and inhibiting tumor cell migration and invasion [39]. Immunomodulator peptides can stimulate human responses and reduce inflammation [40]. In addition, nattokinase, a lytic enzyme produced by *B. subtilis* natto, may play an important role in cardiovascular health through its fibrinolytic properties [7].

Polyketides have a wide spectrum of bioactivity, such as antimicrobial, antitumoral, immunosuppressive, and many antagonistic abilities, and can consequently be used in the human health sector. For instance, dihydroisocoumarins exhibit strong activity against *Helicobacter pylori* [41].

EPS possesses multiple biological functions, such as anticancer, antimicrobial, anti-inflammatory, and immunostimulant activities, and shows prebiotic effects in enhancing probiotic capacity in the gut by acting as protective agents for intestinal health [29].

Organic acids such as dipicolinic acid and L-lactic acid are beneficial for human health by playing an anti-blood coagulation role [42] and an antimicrobe role [43], respectively. Terpenoids, also known as isoprenoids, are represented by some vitamins, such as metaquinone-7 or vitamin K2, and antioxidants (e.g., carotenoids) are, for instance, potential nutraceuticals, while isopentenol may be a potential therapeutic agent in malaria and cancer treatment [31].

Volatile organic and inorganic metabolites have a wide spectrum of antimicrobial activities against several human and plant pathogens in both prevention and treatment actions, for instance, against Candida albicans, one of the most common deep pathogenic fungi [44]. Interestingly, nitric oxide compounds can play a role in human longevity and stress resistance enhancement [5].

B. subtilis is also recognized as a plant growth promoter [45] and biocontrol agent, as well as a biofertilizer, through nitrogen fixation, phosphate solubilization, mitigation of ammonia emission, and improvement of nutrient availability in the soil. As plant growth promotor rhizobacteria (PGPR), *B. subtilis* produces phytohormones (e.g., indole-3-acetic acid), fixing atmospheric N via nitrogenase activity and solubilizing phosphorus [8]. Owing to metabolite production, including antimicrobial peptides (AMPs), cellulolytic and chitinase activity enzymes, VOCs, EPS, and quorum quenching compounds, *B. subtilis* is recognized as a biocontrol agent via direct and indirect mechanisms such as plant growth-promoting metabolites, inducing systemic resistance (ISR), forming biofilm, and inhibiting deleterious phytopathogens.

Finally, *B. subtilis* is an excellent bioremediating agent of contaminated soil, wastewater [46], and even air when associated with plants [47]. It can be used as a detoxifying and degrading agent of heavy metals [48, 49] and contaminant hydrocarbons [50] thanks to enzymes, biosurfactants, and biodegradative compounds. These compounds convert complex organic pollutants into less or non-toxic compounds. **Table 1** lists some examples of important biomolecules produced by *B. subtilis* and their functionalities, as well as the possible roles in One Health.

Health applications	Category	Compounds	Roles	Ref.
Human health prevention and treatment	Enzyme Vitamin Organic acid Amino acid Oligosaccharide Inorganic compound	*Nattokinase* *Menaquinone-7* *Dipicolinic acid* *L-ornithine* *2′-fucosyllactose* *Nitric oxide*	*Fibrinolytic activity* *Anti-arterial calcification* *Anti-blood coagulation* *Anti-obesity* *Prebiotic activity* *Longevity and stress resistance enhancer*	[20] [51] [42] [21] [28] [33]
Animal growth and protection	Enzyme Lipopeptide EPS	*Protease* *Surfactin* *ß-glucan*	*Shrimp growth performance* *Antimicrobe* *Immunostimulant in tilapia*	[52] [53] [54]
Plant growth and protection	Enzyme Organic acid	*Cellulases* *Indole-3-acetic acid*	*Plant defense against pathogens* *Phytohormone (PGPR)*	[8] [55]
Soil and environmental health	Enzymes Polyamino acid Lipopeptide	*Chitinase* *Poly-Υ- glutamic acid* *Surfactin*	*Bioremediation* *Biofertilizer, biochelator* *Bioremediation*	[8] [48] [53]

EPS: Exopolysaccharides; PGPR: Plant Growth-Promoting Rhizobacteria.

Table 1.
Representative biomolecules excreted by B. subtilis *and their potent roles in One Health.*

3. Properties of *B. subtilis* relevant to One Health

B. subtilis is a Gram-positive, rod-shaped bacterium known for its remarkable resilience and adaptability. Its ability to form endospores allows it to endure extreme environmental conditions, making it a common inhabitant of soil, as well as the gastrointestinal tracts of both humans and animals. This resilience, combined with its diverse metabolic capabilities, positions *B. subtilis* as a key player in the concept of One Health, which underscores the interconnectedness of human, animal, plant, and environmental health [56]. As a highly adaptable organism, *B. subtilis* can thrive in a variety of environments, including soil, water, and the gastrointestinal systems of humans and animals. It is also capable of withstanding extreme conditions such as high temperatures, desiccation, and nutrient deprivation. This adaptability is primarily due to its endospore-forming ability, metabolic flexibility, and capacity to interact with various ecosystems. Additionally, *B. subtilis* is recognized for its safety and low pathogenicity, making it an excellent candidate for a wide range of applications in human and animal health [36]. Its long history of use in food, probiotics, and agriculture, along with its regulatory approvals, highlights its status as a beneficial microorganism [57]. Known for its effectiveness as a probiotic, *B. subtilis* survives harsh gastrointestinal environments, influences gut microbiota, and boosts immune responses [58]. Extensive research has demonstrated its benefits in promoting digestive health, inhibiting pathogens, and regulating immune functions in both humans and animals [59].

3.1 Antimicrobial properties

The Bacillus genus is well-known for its production of a diverse array of antimicrobial peptides (AMPs), positioning it as a promising source for the discovery of novel inhibitory compounds [60]. It is estimated that approximately 4–5% of the genetic material in *B. subtilis* strains is dedicated to the synthesis of antimicrobial compounds (AMCs), primarily in the form of AMPs [4]. The production of these bioactive metabolites is heavily dependent on the strain characteristics and the growth of medium conditions. Factors such as the composition of the medium, pH, temperature, and cultivation duration are pivotal in shaping the antibiotic properties of microorganisms [61]. *B. subtilis* produces a variety of antimicrobial compounds that possess potent antibacterial and antifungal activities. These compounds are essential in inhibiting the growth of pathogenic microorganisms in various environments. A crucial survival mechanism of *B. subtilis* is its ability to form highly resilient endospores. In response to environmental stress such as heat, radiation, desiccation, or nutrient scarcity, the bacterium undergoes sporulation, encapsulating its genetic material within a protective spore coat. These endospores can remain dormant for extended periods and reactivate once conditions become more favorable [62]. Furthermore, *B. subtilis* produces antimicrobial substances, including surfactin and subtilin, which effectively inhibit the growth of harmful pathogens like *Clostridium difficile*, Salmonella, and *Escherichia coli*. This antimicrobial activity prevents infections and maintains a balanced gut microbiome [63]. Lipopeptides produced by *B. subtilis* exhibit strong antimicrobial properties, especially against multidrug-resistant bacteria. Owing to their amphiphilic structure, they reduce the surface tension during cultivation and show significant inhibitory effects against *Enterococcus faecalis, Staphylococcus aureus, Pseudomonas aeruginosa,* and *Escherichia coli* [64].

3.2 Probiotic potential

The robust endospore of *B. subtilis* enables it to survive in the acidic environment of the stomach, allowing it to colonize the gut. Once established, *B. subtilis* plays a crucial role in modulating the gut microbiome by promoting the growth of beneficial bacteria such as Lactobacillus and Bifidobacterium, which support digestive health, alleviate gastrointestinal disorders, and enhance immune responses. *B. subtilis* supplementation can reduce symptoms of irritable bowel syndrome and lower the incidence of diarrhea [57]. *B. subtilis* is naturally present in the gut microbiota of both humans and animals. Surviving stomach acidity in its spore form, it germinates in the intestines and helps maintain gut homeostasis. Studies indicate that *B. subtilis* regulates immune functions, supports beneficial gut flora growth, and inhibits pathogenic microorganisms [65]. Unlike other Bacillus species that may produce harmful toxins, *B. subtilis* is non-pathogenic and does not produce enterotoxins or hemolysins, ensuring its safety [36]. Clinical trials on humans have shown that even at high doses (~10^9 spores or CFU/day), *B. subtilis* strains did not cause infections in healthy individuals, making it a safe choice for probiotic use [66, 67]. Unlike many probiotics that are vulnerable to stomach acidity, the spores of *B. subtilis* are highly resistant to harsh conditions, enabling them to pass through the stomach and germinate in the intestines. *B. subtilis* modulates immune responses by stimulating immunoglobulin A (IgA) production and enhancing the activity of macrophages and dendritic cells, bolstering overall health and improving defenses against infections [68]. For instance, *B. subtilis* KATMIRA1933 demonstrates strong probiotic potential, with notable bile salt tolerance, acid resistance, and antimicrobial activity against oral pathogens. Their non-mutagenic properties and ability to co-aggregate with pathogens further support their safety for use in healthcare and food applications [69]. Its antimicrobial properties, immune modulation, and ability to normalize gut flora make it a strong candidate for clinical applications, particularly in preventing and treating diarrhea [70]. Furthermore, *B. subtilis* natto is gaining recognition as a probiotic in animal nutrition, offering antimicrobial, anti-inflammatory, antioxidant, and immunomodulatory benefits that contribute to animal health and food safety, supporting sustainable livestock production [6].

4. *B. subtilis* applications in One Health

4.1 Human health applications

4.1.1 Probiotic formulations for gut health

B. subtilis has been extensively studied for its probiotic properties, demonstrating resilience due to its ability to form spores that withstand gastric acidity, thereby facilitating effective colonization of the gut [59]. Its probiotic benefits include modulation of gut microbiota, enhancement of nutrient absorption, and mitigation of gastrointestinal disorders such as diarrhea and inflammatory bowel diseases [29]. Furthermore, *B. subtilis* improves intestinal barrier integrity by upregulating tight junction proteins and reducing inflammation [71]. A randomized, double-blind, placebo-controlled trial investigated the gastrointestinal (GI) viability and tolerance of *B. subtilis* R0179 in healthy adults across a dose range of 0.1 to 10 $\times$ 10^9 CFU/day. The results indicated no adverse effects on general wellness or GI function, with a dose-dependent increase in fecal viable counts, confirming the strain's ability to survive passage through the GI tract [72]. Another study assessed the safety and tolerability of *B. subtilis* HU58 in patients with hepatic encephalopathy undergoing lactulose treatment. The probiotic group exhibited a trend toward reduced blood ammonia levels, with a significant decrease observed in individuals with baseline ammonia levels above 60 μg/dL, highlighting its potential in managing hepatic encephalopathy [73]. The effects of a probiotic formulation (MegaDuo™) containing *Bacillus coagulans* SC208 and *B. subtilis* HU58 were evaluated on intestinal permeability and immune markers using in vitro models. Under antibiotic-induced dysbiosis, MegaDuo™ improved gut membrane barrier function and reduced levels of pro-inflammatory cytokines TNFα and IL-6. Notably, these benefits were observed after 2 weeks of treatment, whereas no significant effects were detected under normal conditions [74]. *B. subtilis* plays a beneficial role in inflammatory bowel disease management [75]. For instance, a probiotic formulation containing *B. subtilis* alongside *Streptococcus thermophilus*, *Lactobacillus casei*, *Bifidobacterium breve*, and *Bifidobacterium animalis* subsp. lactis in an experimental colitis model showed comparable efficacy to Vivomixx®, reducing colitis symptoms, lowering pro-inflammatory cytokines (IL-6, TNF-α), and increasing anti-inflammatory markers (IL-10) and regulatory T cells (Tregs).

4.1.2 Antibacterial and anti-inflammatory properties

Lipopeptides from *B. subtilis* exhibit potent antimicrobial activity against pathogenic bacteria, including *Escherichia coli*, *Clostridium difficile*, and *Salmonella* spp., by disrupting microbial membranes and inhibiting pathogen colonization [76]. In addition to its direct antimicrobial properties, *B. subtilis* exerts immunomodulatory effects by regulating cytokine production, thereby mitigating inflammatory responses in conditions such as ulcerative colitis and Crohn's disease [77]. A study evaluating the functional properties of various *B. subtilis* strains demonstrated their anti-inflammatory, antioxidant, and antimicrobial activities and effectively inhibited the growth of skin pathogens, underscoring their potential as a functional probiotic material [78]. A comparative study assessed the effects of *Bacillus licheniformis* and *B. subtilis* on IPEC-J2 cells challenged with *E. coli* or *Salmonella Typhimurium*. Both strains demonstrated anti-inflammatory and antioxidant effects, as well as inhibited pathogen adhesion, although they had minimal impact on paracellular permeability. These findings suggest that *Bacillus* species could enhance probiotic efficacy in multispecies formulations [79].

4.1.3 Potential in functional foods and therapeutic agents

B. subtilis has been widely integrated into functional foods and dietary supplements due to its ability to produce beneficial enzymes, vitamins, and bioactive compounds. Fermented foods containing *B. subtilis* have been linked to improved digestion and immune function, making them valuable components of health-promoting diets [80]. Additionally, *B. subtilis* fermentation enhances the bioavailability of nutrients and bioactive compounds, contributing to the overall nutritional value of functional foods. A study on soybean fermentation using protease-producing *B. subtilis* strains (MTCC5480 and MTCC1747) from the Sikkim Himalayan region demonstrated significant improvements in antioxidant activity. The fermentation process increased radical scavenging activity, total antioxidant capacity, and reduced power, attributed to enhanced protein hydrolysis, elevated levels of free phenolics, and the release of amino acids such as proline and tyrosine. Furthermore, the fermented by-products exhibited strain-specific antioxidant properties, indicating their potential as functional food and feed additives with health benefits [81]. Beyond its role in food fermentation, *B. subtilis* has garnered interest in biotechnology due to its potential as a delivery system for therapeutic agents, including vaccines and recombinant proteins. Engineered *B. subtilis* strains are being actively investigated for their ability to express and deliver antigens in oral vaccination strategies, offering a promising approach for mucosal immunization [82]. The robust spore-forming nature of *B. subtilis* enhances its stability and viability, making it an attractive candidate for the development of oral vaccine platforms and biologics.

4.2 Animal health applications

4.2.1 Role in livestock health in improving growth and immunity

The use of *B. subtilis*-based probiotics in animal husbandry has gained significant attention as a sustainable alternative to antibiotic growth promoters. Research in poultry and livestock has demonstrated that dietary supplementation with *B. subtilis* enhances feed conversion efficiency, promotes a balanced gut microbiota, and strengthens immune responses, thereby increasing resistance to enteric pathogens [83]. By stimulating the production of short-chain fatty acids (SCFAs) and reducing intestinal inflammation, *B. subtilis* contributes to improved gut health and reduced dependency on antibiotics in farmed animals.

As a Gram-positive, facultative aerobic bacterium recognized as generally safe, *B. subtilis* plays a crucial role in livestock management. Its probiotic functions include modulation of the gut microbiome, enhancement of immunity, inhibition of pathogenic microorganisms, and secretion of bioactive compounds that support gastrointestinal health and disease resistance. Additionally, *B. subtilis* spores have been explored as vaccine carriers for antigen delivery, further expanding their applications in veterinary medicine [84]. A six-week feeding trial in broilers supplemented with *B. subtilis* BYS2 resulted in a 17.19% increase in body weight, improved intestinal morphology, enhanced immunity (elevated IgG and IgM levels), and greater resistance to Escherichia coli and Newcastle virus infections, leading to improved survival rates [85]. In rabbits, dietary supplementation with *B. subtilis* improved growth performance, strengthened immune responses (higher IgG and IgA levels), and enhanced disease resistance against E. coli. The study suggested that *B. subtilis* supplementation might boost innate immunity through β-defensin induction [47].

A 21-day feeding trial in chickens demonstrated that *B. subtilis* supplementation led to improved growth, immune responses (increased IgA and IgM levels), and intestinal health, as evidenced by increased villus height and a well-balanced microbiota. Additionally, *B. subtilis* improved disease resistance following an E. coli challenge, potentially through Toll-like receptor 4 (TLR4) activation [86]. In broilers, supplementation with *B. subtilis* (0.1 g/kg diet) resulted in improved body weight and feeding conversion ratios. Treated birds also exhibited enhanced immune responses, including higher antibody titers against Newcastle disease, improved lymphoid organ development, and better gut morphology [87].

4.2.2 Use in veterinary probiotics and feed additives

The inclusion of *B. subtilis* in animal feed has been widely explored as a probiotic strategy to improve digestion, prevent gastrointestinal infections, and enhance overall animal health. The bacterium contributes to gut homeostasis by modulating microbiota, promoting beneficial bacterial populations, and inhibiting pathogenic microorganisms. Additionally, *B. subtilis* aids in breaking down indigestible feed components, such as fiber and non-starch polysaccharides, thereby improving nutrient bioavailability and supporting intestinal health in livestock [88]. A study evaluating broiler diets containing both *B. subtilis* and an antimicrobial growth promoter (AGP) reported improved feed conversion efficiency and weight gain compared to diets with either *B. subtilis* or AGP alone, though carcass yield remained unaffected [89]. Supplementation with *B. subtilis* C-3102 spores in broilers, for instance, improved growth performance, feed efficiency, and nutrient digestibility, while also increasing Lactobacillus populations and reducing *Escherichia coli* and Salmonella levels in the gut. Additionally, this probiotic reduced ammonia emissions, demonstrating its potential for improving both animal health and environmental sustainability [90]. Another strain, *B. subtilis* AMS6, isolated from fermented soybeans, exhibited antibacterial activity against *Salmonella enterica*. Its cellulolytic activity suggests a potential role in enhancing fiber digestion and gut health when used as an animal feed additive [91]. A study evaluating *B. subtilis* RBT-7/32 and *B. licheniformis* RBT-11/17 as probiotic feed additives found both strains to exhibit strong antagonistic activity against *E. coli* and *Staphylococcus aureus*. Additionally, *B. subtilis* RBT-7/32 demonstrated increased cellulolytic and amylolytic activity. Both strains showed high spore survivability and resistance to veterinary antibiotics, highlighting their potential for use in livestock nutrition [92]. In aquaculture, *B. subtilis* has been utilized to improve water quality, enhance the immune response of fish and shrimp, and reduce the incidence of bacterial diseases [93]. The probiotic modulates gut microbiota, increases nutrient utilization efficiency, and supports intestinal barrier function in aquatic species. Its ability to degrade organic matter and promote biofloc formation further enhances water quality, thereby creating a more sustainable and disease-resistant environment [88].

4.3 Agricultural applications

4.3.1 Biocontrol agent against plant pathogens

B. subtilis is a well-established biological control agent known for its ability to suppress plant pathogens through multiple mechanisms, including competition for nutrients and space, the induction of systemic resistance, and the production of antimicrobial lipopeptides [94]. Its application in agriculture has been effective in managing fungal pathogens such as Fusarium, Rhizoctonia, and Botrytis, reducing crop losses while minimizing reliance on chemical pesticides. Additionally, *B. subtilis* colonizes plant roots and forms biofilms, creating a protective barrier against infections. *B. subtilis* has been shown to suppress plant pathogens through plant growth promotion, antibiosis, and induced systemic resistance, providing an eco-friendly alternative to synthetic pesticides [95]. A strain of *B. subtilis* isolated from the rhizosphere of chili plants exhibited, for instance, strong antagonistic activity against *Colletotrichum gloeosporioides* through the production of mycolytic enzymes. It significantly reduced fungal growth and improved chili seed germination, demonstrating the potential for biocontrol applications [96]. *B. subtilis* strains isolated from *Zea mays* exhibited over 40% in vitro inhibition of Botrytis cinerea, primarily through lipopeptide production, siderophore activity, and biofilm formation. These strains also promoted maize growth and reduced *B. cinerea* infection in *Phaseolus vulgaris* [97]. *B. subtilis* strains AI01 and AI03, isolated from the eggplant rhizosphere, exhibited strong antagonistic activity against *Fusarium solani*. They inhibited multiple fungal pathogens, produced antifungal metabolites and plant growth-promoting compounds, and reduced wilt incidence by up to 72% in sterilized soil, highlighting their potential as bioinoculants for sustainable disease management [98]. Six *B. subtilis* strains isolated from natural environments in China exhibited over 50% biocontrol efficacy against *Ralstonia solanacearum* in tomato plants. These strains formed robust biofilms on plant roots, demonstrating strong antagonistic activity. Biofilm formation and matrix production were crucial for plant protection, emphasizing their role in bacterial colonization and disease suppression [99].

4.3.2 Fertilizer production and plant growth promotion

As a plant growth-promoting rhizobacterium (PGPR), *B. subtilis* enhances plant root development by producing phytohormones such as indole-3-acetic acid (IAA) and solubilizing phosphorus, thereby increasing nutrient availability for plants [100]. Additionally, its nitrogen-fixing capabilities contribute to soil fertility, making it an essential component of sustainable agricultural practices. The application of *B. subtilis*-based biofertilizers has been associated with improved crop yield, enhanced stress tolerance, and reduced dependency on chemical fertilizers. *B. subtilis* enhances plant growth and stress tolerance through direct and indirect biocontrol mechanisms. It produces secondary metabolites, enzymes, and hormones that suppress pathogens while inducing systemic resistance. Additionally, it improves soil nutrient availability and promotes root colonization, making it a valuable biofertilizer and biopesticide [101]. For instance, a biofertilizer (BOF) containing *B. subtilis* F2 significantly enhanced strawberry plant growth, nutrient accumulation, and peroxidase activity. BOF also altered the rhizosphere microbial community's β-diversity, suggesting strain F2 played a crucial role in plant health improvement [102]. Another strain (*B. subtilis* L2) significantly improved ginger growth by increasing plant height, leaf length, number of leaves, and chlorophyll content. Inoculation enhanced physiological properties, supporting its potential as a promising biofertilizer for ginger cultivation [103]. Field trials in Tajikistan showed that *B. subtilis* FZB 24® increased cotton yield by up to 30% compared to conventional NPK fertilizer. The treatment enhanced root growth and phosphorus mobilization, demonstrating its potential as an eco-friendly alternative to chemical fertilizers [104]. *B. subtilis*, alone or in combination with nutrients, effectively controlled early blight in tomatoes (67–83%) and enhanced plant growth (20–77%). The treatment boosted phenolic content and defensive enzyme activity, highlighting its synergistic effect with NPK and Zn (2X) in disease management and plant health improvement [105].

4.4 Environmental applications

4.4.1 Bioremediation of environmental pollutants

The application of *B. subtilis* in environmental biotechnology has garnered attention due to its capacity to degrade hydrocarbons and detoxify heavy metals. It plays a crucial role in breaking down oil spills, pesticide residues, and industrial pollutants through enzymatic biodegradation [106]. The production of biosurfactants further enhances its bioremediation potential by aiding in the emulsification and breakdown of hydrophobic contaminants, making them more accessible for microbial degradation. *B. subtilis* isolated from a polymer dump site in Chennai, India, degraded 80% of crude oil and reduced viscosity by 60% within 10 days. Its biosurfactant production, high emulsification efficiency, and stability under extreme conditions highlight its potential for oil spill remediation [107]. *B. subtilis*, widely utilized in bioengineering and biotechnology, forms robust biofilms and spores that enhance its resilience and versatility. These biofilms, composed of exopolysaccharides, proteins, extracellular DNA, and poly-γ-glutamic acid, support applications in bioremediation, biosensing, and biocatalysis. Advances in synthetic biology have enabled the engineering of *B. subtilis* biofilms for self-regenerating and environmentally responsive biomaterials, broadening their utility in sustainable technologies [108]. Biosurfactant concentrations of 19–19.5 mg/kg stimulated hydrocarbon-degrading microbial populations and accelerated aliphatic hydrocarbon degradation. However, its effect on aromatic hydrocarbon degradation was limited [109]. Two *B. subtilis* strains (M16K and M19F) demonstrated simultaneous hydrocarbon degradation and heavy metal (Co^{2+} and Ni^{2+}) removal in contaminated environments. These strains achieved >94% crude oil and >85% phenanthrene degradation while concurrently detoxifying heavy metals within 18–28 days. This study represents the first report of metal-resistant *B. subtilis* strains with dual bioremediation capabilities in sub-Saharan Africa, underscoring their potential for multi-polluted site restoration [110].

4.4.2 Waste management and decomposition

B. subtilis contributes significantly to organic waste degradation by producing cellulases and proteases that accelerate biodegradation processes. Its application in composting enhances nutrient cycling, improves soil fertility, and reduces environmental waste accumulation [111]. Additionally, its ability to break down agricultural residues and convert organic matter into biofertilizers supports sustainable waste management practices. Inoculating compost with *B. subtilis* at a 2% concentration enhanced fermentation but suppressed the synthesis of total organic carbon and humus. In contrast, a 0.5% inoculation significantly improved carbon humification, resulting in a 12.5% increase in total organic carbon and a 20.2% increase in humic substances compared to the 2% treatment [112]. Parameters such as pH and microbial metabolism played key roles in carbon sequestration during composting. In a sequencing batch reactor (SBR), *B. subtilis* improved sludge treatment in recirculating aquaculture systems (RAS). Biofloc crude protein content increased by 23.97% over the control, while removal rates of dissolved inorganic nitrogen (1.17×), total organic nitrogen (1.71×), and dissolved organic carbon (1.95×) were significantly enhanced. Floc volume after 5 minutes reached 22.67% at 19 days [113]. India faces significant post-harvest losses, with approximately 30% of fruit and vegetable production wasted annually. A study exploring *B. subtilis* isolated from pomegranate peel demonstrated its potential as a plant growth-promoting rhizobacterium (PGPR) for agricultural waste management. Treated wheat exhibited increased yield, while microgreens showed higher phenol and antioxidant levels, highlighting *B. subtilis* as a biofertilizer for sustainable agriculture [114]. Solid waste management, particularly concerning petroleum-based plastic and fish solid waste (FSW), remains a global challenge. *B. subtilis* strain KP172548 was shown to convert FSW extract into 1.62 g/L of polyhydroxybutyrate (PHB), a biodegradable biopolymer. The PHB was biocompatible, suggesting its potential as an eco-friendly alternative to conventional plastics [115].

5. Safety and regulation aspects

B. subtilis has a long history of safe use in food fermentation and as a probiotic. Strains such as *B. subtilis* DE111 have been administered in doses up to 10 billion colony-forming units daily for periods ranging from 2 to 8 weeks without adverse effects [59]. It is approved for use in food in certain European countries [116] and is also naturally present in traditional Asian foods such as natto and kimchi [66, 117]. This safety profile has led to its recognition as a safe organism in various applications, including food production and dietary supplementation [116]. In the U.S., the Food and Drug Administration (FDA) grants Generally Recognized As Safe (GRAS) status to *B. subtilis* strains through assessments that include strain characterization, genome sequencing, screening for undesirable attributes and metabolites, and experimental safety evaluations conducted in appropriately designed studies. At least five GRAS notifications for *B. subtilis* in food applications have been approved without questions from the FDA [118].

European Food Safety Authority (EFSA) has established the Qualified Presumption of Safety (QPS) approach to assess the safety of microorganisms. To meet QPS status requirements, any new *B. subtilis* strain must be identified at both the strain and species levels, be free of transferable antimicrobial resistance, and exhibit no toxigenic activity [67]. *B. subtilis* is included in the list of QPS-recommended microorganisms and considered to have QPS status when used as an animal feed additive, owing to its lack of toxigenic activity [119].

Several studies have assessed the safety of *B. subtilis* strains for human consumption, including both in vitro and clinical evaluations. For example, *B. subtilis* CU1 was shown to be free of antibiotic resistance and caused no physiological or biological issues in adults consuming 2 x 10^9 spores per day for 40 days [67]. *B. subtilis* MB40 was also found to be safe at a daily intake of 2.6 x 10^{11} spores/day for a 70 kg adult [66].

As a feed additive, EFSA's safety evaluation did not reveal any toxigenic activity or antibiotic resistance in *B. subtilis*, and it is therefore considered safe for animals [120, 121]. Moreover, *B. subtilis* strains have been approved by the Environmental Protection Agency (EPA) as biocides and are exempt from tolerance limits in food crops, as they are not considered toxic or pathogenic to humans, animals, or plants [122].

However, the use of *Bacillus* species raises safety concerns due to the potential production of enterotoxins and emetic toxins, which are strain-specific [123]. Therefore, it is crucial to assess and confirm the safety of potential probiotics at a strain level prior to their use. Adhering to regulatory standards and ensuring safety are critical for guaranteeing the safety of probiotics. These regulations are guided by the criteria set by national authorities, including the European Food Safety Authority (EFSA), the U.S. Food and Drug Administration (FDA), and the Canadian Natural and Non-Prescription Health Products Directorate [124].

Emerging concerns about the safety of probiotics, particularly their potential risks for immunocompromised individuals, underline the need for in-depth safety studies [125]. Recommendations for future regulatory frameworks have been proposed, emphasizing the importance of assessing both acute and long-term safety. Probiotics intended for specific patient populations should undergo rigorous testing to ensure they meet quality standards, ideally verified by an independent third party. Additional research is essential to fill existing knowledge gaps, including identifying the most suitable animal models for safety testing, assessing the potential transfer of antibiotic resistance genes, and exploring the effects of probiotics on microbiomes, drug interactions, and colonization [126].

6. Conclusion

B. subtilis is a bacterial species with immense potential for producing a high diversity of bioactive compounds, ranging from the simple organic and inorganic metabolites to more complex systems such as nanoparticles and vesicles. These compounds serve a variety of properties and functions. Recognized as safe, *B. subtilis* is a promising natural candidate for the One Health approach, which seeks to optimize the health of people, animals, plants, and the environment. The resilience and adaptability of *B. subtilis* make it a highly valuable microorganism with diverse applications across biotechnology, agriculture, and human health. Its ability to withstand extreme conditions and colonize a wide range of environments—from soil to the gastrointestinal tracts of humans and animals—highlights its essential role in maintaining ecosystem stability. In human and animal health, *B. subtilis* demonstrates significant probiotic potential, offering health benefits for both the prevention and treatment of various diseases. In agriculture, *B. subtilis* plays a crucial role as a biocontrol agent and biofertilizer, promoting plant growth, enhancing soil fertility, and reducing the need for chemical pesticides and fertilizers. As biotechnological advancements progress, the range of *B. subtilis* applications is expected to expand, providing innovative solutions for global health, food security, and environmental sustainability. Future research should focus on optimizing microbial formulations, utilizing genetic engineering for strain improvement, and integrating *B. subtilis* into precision agriculture, sustainable livestock production, and large-scale environmental restoration projects. By leveraging its natural capabilities, future innovations could enhance public health, promote resilient food systems, and contribute to a more sustainable world.

Acknowledgements

HR was partially funded by the Horizon Europe Research innovation program through URBANE (grant n° 101059232) and CONSERWA (grant n°101081802).

Conflict of interest

The authors declare no conflict of interest.

Author details

Hary Razafindralambo[1,2*], Vijayaram Seerengaraj[2,3] and Holy Rabetafika[2]

1 TERRA Teaching and Research Unit, Gembloux Agro-Bio Tech, University of Liege, Belgium

2 ProBioLab, Namur, Belgium

3 Centre for Global Health Research, Saveetha University, Thandalam, India

*Address all correspondence to: h.razafindralambo@uliege.be

References

[1] Hoque N, Faisal G, Chowdhury F, et al. The Urgency of Wider Adoption of One Health Approach for the Prevention of a Future Pandemic. 2022. Available from: https://acquire.cqu.edu.au/articles/journal_contribution/The_urgency_of_wider_adoption_of_one_health_approach_for_the_prevention_of_a_future_pandemic/25044212 [Accessed: March 6, 2025]

[2] Pepoyan A, Tsaturyan V, Manukyan V, et al. Novel probiotic *Lactiplantibacillus plantarum* str. ZPZ as a possible candidate for "one health" probiotic. In: Ronzhin A, Kostyaev A, editors. Agriculture Digitalization and Organic Production. Singapore: Springer Nature; 2023. pp. 141-150

[3] Kovács ÁT. *Bacillus subtilis*. Trends in Microbiology. 2019;**27**:724-725

[4] Caulier S, Nannan C, Gillis A, et al. Overview of the antimicrobial compounds produced by members of the *Bacillus subtilis* group. Frontiers in Microbiology. 2019;**10**:302

[5] Ayala FR, Bauman C, Cogliati S, et al. Microbial flora, probiotics, *Bacillus subtilis* and the search for a long and healthy human longevity. Microbial Cell. 2017;**4**:133

[6] Ruiz Sella SRB, Bueno T, de Oliveira AAB, et al. *Bacillus subtilis* natto as a potential probiotic in animal nutrition. Critical Reviews in Biotechnology. 2021;**41**:355-369

[7] Miyazawa T, Abe C, Bhaswant M, et al. Biological functions of compounds from *Bacillus subtilis* and its subspecies. *Bacillus subtilis* natto. Food Bioengineering. 2022;**1**:241-251

[8] Alina SO, Constantinscu F, Petruța CC. Biodiversity of *Bacillus subtilis* group and beneficial traits of bacillus species useful in plant protection. Romanian Biotechnological Letters. 2015;**20**:10737-10750

[9] Mahapatra S, Yadav R, Ramakrishna W. *Bacillus subtilis* impact on plant growth, soil health and environment: Dr. Jekyll and Mr. Hyde. Journal of Applied Microbiology. 2022;**132**:3543-3562

[10] Li Y, Cheng L, Yang B, et al. Remediation of Cd-As-Ni co-contaminated soil by extracellular polymeric substances from *Bacillus subtilis*: Dynamic improvements of soil properties and ecotoxicity. Science of the Total Environment. 2024;**955**:177009

[11] Khan S, Akhtar N, Rehman SU, et al. Iron oxide nanoparticle (Fe3 O4 NPs) synthesized from *B. subtilis* reduced arsenic (as) toxicity in rice (*Oryza sativa L.*) plant. International Journal of Phytoremediation. 2024;**26**:1676-1682

[12] Vijayaram S, Razafindralambo H, Sun Y-Z, et al. Applications of green synthesized metal nanoparticles — A review. Biological Trace Element Research. 2023;**202**:360-386. DOI: 10.1007/s12011-023-03645-9

[13] Su Y, Liu C, Fang H, et al. *Bacillus subtilis*: A universal cell factory for industry, agriculture, biomaterials and medicine. Microbial Cell Factories. 2020;**19**:173

[14] Mohkam M, Nezafat N, Berenjian A, et al. Role of bacillus genus in the production of value-added compounds. In: Islam MT, Rahman M, Pandey P, et al., editors. Bacilli and

Agrobiotechnology. Cham: Springer International Publishing. 2016. pp. 1-33

[15] Iqbal S, Begum F, Rabaan AA, et al. Classification and multifaceted potential of secondary metabolites produced by *Bacillus subtilis* group: A comprehensive review. Molecules. 2023;**28**:927

[16] Kaspar F, Neubauer P, Gimpel M. Bioactive secondary metabolites from *Bacillus subtilis*: A comprehensive review. Journal of Natural Products. 2019;**82**:2038-2053

[17] Yu X, Ai C, Xin L, et al. The siderophore-producing bacterium, *Bacillus subtilis* CAS15, has a biocontrol effect on Fusarium wilt and promotes the growth of pepper. European Journal of Soil Biology. 2011;**47**:138-145

[18] Tareq FS, Lee MA, Lee H-S, et al. Gageostatins A–C, antimicrobial linear lipopeptides from a marine *Bacillus subtilis*. Marine Drugs. 2014;**12**:871-885

[19] Nguyen SLT, Inaoka T, Kimura K. Poly-γ-glutamic acid production by *Bacillus subtilis* (natto) under high salt conditions. Japan Agricultural Research Quarterly: JARQ. 2018;**52**:249-253

[20] Chen H, McGowan EM, Ren N, et al. Nattokinase: A promising alternative in prevention and treatment of cardiovascular diseases. Biomarker Insights. 2018;**13**:1177271918785130

[21] Wang Q, Bao T, Hu M, et al. Efficient Acetoin production in *Bacillus subtilis* by multivariate modular metabolic engineering with spatiotemporal modulation. ACS Sustainable Chemistry and Engineering. 2025;**13**:1927-1936

[22] Cheng H-W, Jiang S, Hu J. Gut-brain axis: Probiotic, *Bacillus subtilis*, prevents aggression via the modification of the central serotonergic system. In: Oral Health by Using Probiotic Products. London, UK: IntechOpen; 2019. Available from: https://www.intechopen.com/chapters/67675 [Accessed: February 23, 2025]

[23] McDaniel R, Ebert-Khosla S, Hopwood DA, et al. Engineered biosynthesis of novel polyketides. Science. 1993;**262**:1546-1550

[24] Yan X, Zhou Y-X, Tang X-X, et al. Macrolactins from marine-derived *Bacillus subtilis* B5 bacteria as inhibitors of inducible nitric oxide and cytokines expression. Marine Drugs. 2016;**14**:195

[25] Um S, Fraimout A, Sapountzis P, et al. The fungus-growing termite macrotermes natalensis harbors bacillaene-producing bacillus sp. that inhibit potentially antagonistic fungi. Scientific Reports. 2013;**3**:3250

[26] Nguyen HT. Advances in microbial exopolysaccharides: Present and future applications. Biomolecules. 2024;**14**:1162

[27] Bersaneti GT, Pan NC, Baldo C, et al. Co-production of Fructooligosaccharides and Levan by Levansucrase from *Bacillus subtilis* natto with potential application in the food industry. Applied Biochemistry and Biotechnology. 2018;**184**:838-851

[28] Zhang Q, Liu Z, Xia H, et al. Engineered *Bacillus subtilis* for the de novo production of 2′-fucosyllactose. Microbial Cell Factories. 2022;**21**:110

[29] Lu S, Na K, Li Y, et al. Bacillus -derived probiotics: Metabolites and mechanisms involved in bacteria–host interactions. Critical Reviews in Food Science and Nutrition. 2024;**64**:1701-1714

[30] Pramastya H, Song Y, Elfahmi EY, et al. Positioning *Bacillus subtilis* as terpenoid cell factory. Journal of Applied Microbiology. 2021;**130**:1839-1856

[31] Withers ST, Gottlieb SS, Lieu B, et al. Identification of Isopentenol biosynthetic genes from *Bacillus subtilis* by a screening method based on Isoprenoid precursor toxicity. Applied and Environmental Microbiology. 2007;**73**:6277-6283

[32] Kai M. Diversity and distribution of volatile secondary metabolites throughout *Bacillus subtilis* isolates. Frontiers in Microbiology. 2020;**11**:559

[33] Gusarov I, Gautier L, Smolentseva O, et al. Bacterial nitric oxide extends the lifespan of C. Elegans. Cell. 2013;**152**:818-830

[34] Zhao X, Yan L, Xu X, et al. Synthesis of silver nanoparticles and its contribution to the capability of *Bacillus subtilis* to deal with polluted waters. Applied Microbiology and Biotechnology. 2019;**103**:6319-6332

[35] Kim S-H, Yehuala GA, Bang WY, et al. Safety evaluation of *Bacillus subtilis* IDCC1101, newly isolated from Cheonggukjang, for industrial applications. Microorganisms. 2022;**10**:2494

[36] Sorokulova IB, Pinchuk IV, Denayrolles M, et al. The safety of two bacillus probiotic strains for human use. Digestive Diseases and Sciences. 2008;**53**:954-963

[37] Hosoi T, Kiuchi K. Natto–a food made by fermenting cooked soybeans with Bacillus subtilis (natto). In: Edward RF editor. Handbook of Fermented Functional Foods. New York: Taylor & Francis Group; 2003. pp. 227-245

[38] Chen C, Xiang JY, Hu W, et al. Identification of key micro-organisms involved in Douchi fermentation by statistical analysis and their use in an experimental fermentation. Journal of Applied Microbiology. 2015;**119**:1324-1334

[39] Zhao H, Yan L, Xu X, et al. Potential of *Bacillus subtilis* lipopeptides in anti-cancer I: Induction of apoptosis and paraptosis and inhibition of autophagy in K562 cells. AMB Express. 2018;**8**:78

[40] Nasseri S, Sharifi M. Therapeutic potential of antimicrobial peptides for wound healing. International Journal of Peptide Research and Therapeutics. 2022;**28**:38

[41] Pinchuk IV, Bressollier P, Sorokulova IB, et al. Amicoumacin antibiotic production and genetic diversity of *Bacillus subtilis* strains isolated from different habitats. Research in Microbiology. 2002;**153**:269-276

[42] Ohsugi T, Ikeda S, Sumi H. Anti-platelet aggregation and anti-blood coagulation activities of dipicolinic acid, a sporal component of *Bacillus subtilis* Natto. Food Science and Technology Research. 2005;**11**:308-310

[43] Poudel P, Tashiro Y, Sakai K. New application of bacillus strains for optically pure L-lactic acid production: General overview and future prospects. Bioscience, Biotechnology, and Biochemistry. 2016;**80**:642-654

[44] Wang W, Zhao J, Zhang Z. Bacillus metabolites: Compounds, identification and anti-*Candida albicans* mechanisms. Microbiology Research. 2022;**13**:972-984

[45] Sansinenea E. *Bacillus spp.*: As plant growth-promoting bacteria. In: Singh HB, Keswani C, Reddy MS, et al., editors. Secondary Metabolites of Plant Growth Promoting Rhizomicroorganisms: Discovery and Applications. Singapore: Springer; 2019. pp. 225-237

[46] Migahed F, Abdelrazak A, Fawzy G. Batch and continuous removal of heavy metals from industrial effluents using

microbial consortia. International journal of Environmental Science and Technology. 2017;**14**:1169-1180

[47] Guo M, Wu F, Hao G, et al. *Bacillus subtilis* improves immunity and disease resistance in rabbits. Frontiers in Immunology. 2017;**8**:354

[48] Pang X, Lei P, Feng X, et al. Poly-γ-glutamic acid, a bio-chelator, alleviates the toxicity of Cd and Pb in the soil and promotes the establishment of healthy *Cucumis sativus L.* seedling. Environmental Science and Pollution Research. 2018;**25**:19975-19988

[49] Mardiyono M, Hidayati N. Bioremediation of chrome heavy metals on metal coating waste with *Bacillus subtilis* bacteria. In: AIP Conference Proceedings. Surakarta, Indonesia: AIP Publishing; 2020. Available from: https://pubs.aip.org/aip/acp/article-abstract/2296/1/020033/724120 [Accessed: February 28, 2025]

[50] Nimrat S, Lookchan S, Boonthai T, et al. Bioremediation of petroleum contaminated soils by lipopeptide producing *Bacillus subtilis* SE1. African Journal of Biotechnology. 2019;**18**:494-501

[51] Mandatori D, Pelusi L, Schiavone V, et al. The dual role of vitamin K2 in "bone-vascular crosstalk": Opposite effects on bone loss and vascular calcification. Nutrients. 2021;**13**:1222

[52] Liu C-H, Chiu C-S, Ho P-L, et al. Improvement in the growth performance of white shrimp, Litopenaeus vannamei, by a protease-producing probiotic, *Bacillus subtilis* E20, from natto. Journal of Applied Microbiology. 2009;**107**:1031-1041

[53] Hamley IW. Lipopeptides: From self-assembly to bioactivity. Chemical Communications. 2015;**51**:8574-8583

[54] Gao T, Wong Y, Ng C, et al. L-lactic acid production by *Bacillus subtilis* MUR1. Bioresource Technology. 2012;**121**:105-110

[55] Shinde SS, Gaonkar VV, Mukadam HM, et al. *Bacillus subtilis*: A Biological Marvel in the Domain of Agriculture and Environmental Science. 2025. Available from: https://www.intechopen.com/online-first/1202535 [Accessed: February 28, 2025]

[56] Ortiz A, Sansinenea E. *Bacillus sp*. as biofertilizers applied in horticultural crops. In: Rakshit A, Meena VS, Fraceto LF, et al., editors. Bio-Inoculants in Horticultural Crops. Sawtson, Cambridge: Woodhead Publishing; 2024. pp. 97-108

[57] Elshaghabee FM, Rokana N, Gulhane RD, et al. Bacillus as potential probiotics: Status, concerns, and future perspectives. Frontiers in Microbiology. 2017;**8**:1490

[58] Freedman KE, Hill JL, Wei Y, et al. Examining the gastrointestinal and immunomodulatory effects of the novel probiotic *Bacillus subtilis* DE111. International Journal of Molecular Sciences. 2021;**22**:2453

[59] Williams N, Weir TL. Spore-based probiotic *Bacillus subtilis*: Current applications in humans and future perspectives. Fermentation. 2024;**10**:78

[60] Sumi CD, Yang BW, Yeo I-C, et al. Antimicrobial peptides of the genus bacillus: A new era for antibiotics. Canadian Journal of Microbiology. 2015;**61**:93-103

[61] Sidorova TM, Asaturova AM, Homyak AI, et al. Optimization of laboratory cultivation conditions for the synthesis of antifungal metabolites by *Bacillus subtilis* strains. Saudi Journal of Biological Sciences. 2020;**27**:1879-1885

[62] Setlow P. Spore resistance properties. Microbiology Spectrum. 2014;**2**:1-14. DOI: 10.1128/microbiolspec.TBS-0003-2012

[63] Golnari M, Bahrami N, Milanian Z, et al. Isolation and characterization of novel bacillus strains with superior probiotic potential: Comparative analysis and safety evaluation. Scientific Reports. 2024;**14**:1457

[64] Fernandes PAV, De AIR, Dos SAFAB, et al. Antimicrobial activity of surfactants produced by *Bacillus subtilis* R14 against multidrug-resistant bacteria. Brazilian Journal of Microbiology. 2007;**38**:704-709

[65] Tam NKM, Uyen NQ, Hong HA, et al. The intestinal life cycle of *Bacillus subtilis* and close relatives. Journal of Bacteriology. 2006;**188**:2692-2700

[66] Spears JL, Kramer R, Nikiforov AI, et al. Safety assessment of *Bacillus subtilis* MB40 for use in foods and dietary supplements. Nutrients. 2021;**13**:733

[67] Lefevre M, Racedo SM, Denayrolles M, et al. Safety assessment of *Bacillus subtilis* CU1 for use as a probiotic in humans. Regulatory Toxicology and Pharmacology. 2017;**83**:54-65

[68] Ghelardi E, Celandroni F, Salvetti S, et al. Survival and persistence of *Bacillus clausii* in the human gastrointestinal tract following oral administration as spore-based probiotic formulation. Journal of Applied Microbiology. 2015;**119**:552-559

[69] AlGburi A, Volski A, Cugini C, et al. Safety properties and probiotic potential of *Bacillus subtilis* KATMIRA1933 and bacillus amyloliquefaciens B-1895. Advances in Microbiology. 2016;**6**:432-452

[70] Suva MA, Sureja VP, Kheni DB. Novel insight on probiotic *Bacillus subtilis*: Mechanism of action and clinical applications. Journal of Current Research in Scientific Medicine. 2016;**2**:65

[71] Dang HT, Tran DM, Phung TTB, et al. Promising clinical and immunological efficacy of *Bacillus clausii* spore probiotics for supportive treatment of persistent diarrhea in children. Scientific Reports. 2024;**14**:6422

[72] Hanifi A, Culpepper T, Mai V, et al. Evaluation of *Bacillus subtilis* R0179 on gastrointestinal viability and general wellness: A randomised, double-blind, placebo-controlled trial in healthy adults. Beneficial Microbes. 2015;**6**:19-28

[73] Yossef S, Clark F, Bubeck SS, et al. An Oral formulation of the probiotic, *Bacillus subtilis* HU58, was safe and well tolerated in a pilot study of patients with hepatic encephalopathy. Evidence-based Complementary and Alternative Medicine. 2020;**2020**:1463108

[74] Marzorati M, Van den Abbeele P, Bubeck SS, et al. *Bacillus subtilis* HU58 and Bacillus coagulans SC208 probiotics reduced the effects of antibiotic-induced gut microbiome dysbiosis in an M-SHIME® model. Microorganisms. 2020;**8**:1028

[75] Biagioli M, Carino A, Di Giorgio C, et al. Discovery of a novel multi-strains probiotic formulation with improved efficacy toward intestinal inflammation. Nutrients. 2020;**12**:1945

[76] Corona R, Bontà V, Baccigalupi L, et al. Probiotic spores of *Shouchella clausii* SF174 and displayed bromelain show beneficial additive potential. International Journal of Molecular Sciences. 2025;**26**:942

[77] Xie H, Yu T, Zhou Q, et al. Comparative evaluation of spores and vegetative forms of *Bacillus subtilis*

and bacillus licheniformis on probiotic functionality In vitro and In vivo. Probiotics and Antimicrobial Proteins. 2024. DOI: 10.1007/s12602-024-10407-z

[78] Jung H-S, Lee H-W, Kim K-T, et al. Anti-inflammatory, antioxidant effects, and antimicrobial effect of *Bacillus subtilis* P223. Food Science and Biotechnology. 2024;**33**:2179-2187

[79] Palkovicsné Pézsa N, Kovács D, Rácz B, et al. Effects of bacillus licheniformis and *Bacillus subtilis* on gut barrier function, proinflammatory response, ROS production and pathogen inhibition properties in IPEC-J2—Escherichia coli/salmonella typhimurium co-culture. Microorganisms. 2022;**10**:936

[80] Sultana MS, Khatun M, Rahman A. Antimicrobial activities and probiotic properties of bacillus sp. strains isolated from fermented cooked rice. Microbiology and Biotechnology Letters. 2024;**52**:288-297

[81] Sanjukta S, Rai AK, Muhammed A, et al. Enhancement of antioxidant properties of two soybean varieties of Sikkim Himalayan region by proteolytic *Bacillus subtilis* fermentation. Journal of Functional Foods. 2015;**14**:650-658

[82] Ghosh T. Recent advances in the probiotic application of the bacillus as a potential candidate in the sustainable development of aquaculture. Aquaculture. 2024;**594**:741432

[83] Cai Y, Xiao C, Tian B, et al. Dietary probiotic based on a dual-strain *Bacillus subtilis* improves immunity, intestinal health, and growth performance of broiler chickens. Journal of Animal Science. 2024;**102**:skae183

[84] Yuan C, Ji X, Zhang Y, et al. Important role of *Bacillus subtilis* as a probiotic and vaccine carrier in animal health maintenance. World Journal of Microbiology and Biotechnology. 2024;**40**:268

[85] Dong Y, Li R, Liu Y, et al. Benefit of dietary supplementation with *Bacillus subtilis* BYS2 on growth performance, immune response, and disease resistance of broilers. Probiotics and Antimicrobial Proteins. 2020;**12**:1385-1397

[86] Guo M, Li M, Zhang C, et al. Dietary administration of the *Bacillus subtilis* enhances immune responses and disease resistance in chickens. Frontiers in Microbiology. 2020;**11**:1768

[87] Sikandar A, Zaneb H, Younus M, et al. Growth performance, immune status and organ morphometry in broilers fed *Bacillus subtilis*-supplemented diet. South African Journal of Animal Science. 2017;**47**:378-388

[88] Muthu CM, Vickram AS, Sowndharya BB, et al. A comprehensive review on the utilization of probiotics in aquaculture towards sustainable shrimp farming. Fish and Shellfish Immunology. 2024;**147**:109459

[89] Mingmongkolchai S, Panbangred W. Bacillus probiotics: An alternative to antibiotics for livestock production. Journal of Applied Microbiology. 2018;**124**:1334-1346

[90] Jeong JS, Kim IH. Effect of *Bacillus subtilis* C-3102 spores as a probiotic feed supplement on growth performance, noxious gas emission, and intestinal microflora in broilers. Poultry Science. 2014;**93**:3097-3103

[91] Manhar AK, Bashir Y, Saikia D, et al. Cellulolytic potential of probiotic *Bacillus subtilis* AMS6 isolated from traditional fermented soybean (Churpi): An in-vitro study with regards to application as an

animal feed additive. Microbiological Research. 2016;**186**:62-70

[92] Yaderets V, Karpova N, Glagoleva E, et al. *Bacillus subtilis* RBT-7/32 and bacillus licheniformis RBT-11/17 as new promising strains for use in probiotic feed additives. Microorganisms. 2023;**11**:2729

[93] Hai NV. The use of probiotics in aquaculture. Journal of Applied Microbiology. 2015;**119**:917-935

[94] Shaheb MR, Islam MT, Sarker A, et al. Biofertilizers: Catalysts for enhancing soil and plant health in pursuit of sustainable agriculture. In: Dheeman S, Islam MT, Egamberdieva D, et al., editors. Soil Bacteria. Singapore: Springer Nature; 2024. pp. 3-41

[95] Wang XQ, Zhao DL, Shen LL, et al. Application and mechanisms of *Bacillus subtilis* in biological control of plant disease. In: Meena VS, editor. Role of Rhizospheric Microbes in Soil. Singapore: Springer; 2018. pp. 225-250

[96] Ashwini N, Srividya S. Potentiality of *Bacillus subtilis* as biocontrol agent for management of anthracnose disease of chilli caused by *Colletotrichum gloeosporioides* OGC1. 3 Biotech. 2014;**4**:127-136

[97] Moustafa HE, Abo-Zaid GA, Abd-Elsalam HE, et al. Antagonistic and inhibitory effect of *Bacillus subtilis* against certain plant pathogenic fungi. I. Biotechnology. 2009;**8**:53-61

[98] Saha D, Purkayastha GD, Ghosh A, et al. Isolation and characterization of two new *Bacillus subtilis* strains from the rhizosphere of eggplant as potential biocontrol agents. Journal of Plant Pathology. 2012;**94**:109-118

[99] Chen Y, Yan F, Chai Y, et al. Biocontrol of tomato wilt disease by *Bacillus subtilis* isolates from natural environments depends on conserved genes mediating biofilm formation. Environmental Microbiology. 2013;**15**:848-864

[100] Din UMM, Batool A, Ashraf RS, et al. Green synthesis and characterization of biologically synthesized and antibiotic-conjugated silver nanoparticles followed by post-synthesis assessment for antibacterial and antioxidant applications. ACS Omega. 2024;**9**:18909-18921

[101] Hashem A, Tabassum B, Abd_Allah EF. *Bacillus subtilis*: A plant-growth promoting rhizobacterium that also impacts biotic stress. Saudi Journal of Biological Sciences. 2019;**26**:1291-1297

[102] Liu L, Li X, Li T, et al. Bio-organic fertilizer with *Bacillus subtilis* F2 promotes strawberry plant growth and changes Rhizosphere microbial community. Journal of Soil Science and Plant Nutrition. 2022;**22**:3045-3055

[103] Jabborova D, Enakiev Y, Sulaymanov K, et al. Plant growth promoting bacteria *Bacillus subtilis* promote growth and physiological parameters of Zingiber officinale roscoe. Plant Science Today. 2021;**8**:66-71

[104] Yao AV, Bochow H, Karimov S, et al. Effect of FZB 24® *Bacillus subtilis* as a biofertilizer on cotton yields in field tests. Archives of Phytopathology and Plant Protection. 2006;**39**:323-328

[105] Awan ZA, Shoaib A. Combating early blight infection by employing *Bacillus subtilis* in combination with plant fertilizers. Current Plant Biology. 2019;**20**:100125

[106] Muñoz AJ, Espínola F, Ruiz E, et al. Biocidal and synergistic effect of three types of biologically synthesised

silver/silver chloride nanoparticles. World Journal of Microbiology and Biotechnology. 2024;**40**:18

[107] Sakthipriya N, Doble M, Sangwai JS. Bioremediation of coastal and marine pollution due to crude oil using a microorganism *Bacillus subtilis*. Procedia Engineering. 2015;**116**:213-220

[108] Mohsin MZ, Omer R, Huang J, et al. Advances in engineered *Bacillus subtilis* biofilms and spores, and their applications in bioremediation, biocatalysis, and biomaterials. Synthetic and Systems Biotechnology. 2021;**6**:180-191

[109] Cubitto MA, Morán AC, Commendatore M, et al. Effects of *Bacillus subtilis* O9 biosurfactant on the bioremediation of crude oil-polluted soils. Biodegradation. 2004;**15**:281-287

[110] Oyetibo GO, Chien M-F, Ikeda-Ohtsubo W, et al. Biodegradation of crude oil and phenanthrene by heavy metal resistant *Bacillus subtilis* isolated from a multi-polluted industrial wastewater creek. International Biodeterioration and Biodegradation. 2017;**120**:143-151

[111] Fadiji AE, Xiong C, Egidi E, et al. Formulation challenges associated with microbial biofertilizers in sustainable agriculture and paths forward. Journal of Sustainable Agriculture and Environment. 2024;**3**:e70006

[112] Duan M, Zhang Y, Zhou B, et al. Effects of *Bacillus subtilis* on carbon components and microbial functional metabolism during cow manure–straw composting. Bioresource Technology. 2020;**303**:122868

[113] Lu L, Tan H, Luo G, et al. The effects of *Bacillus subtilis* on nitrogen recycling from aquaculture solid waste using heterotrophic nitrogen assimilation in sequencing batch reactors. Bioresource Technology. 2012;**124**:180-185

[114] Ravichandran M, Samiappan SC, Rangaraj S, et al. Nanoemulsion formulations with plant growth promoting rhizobacteria (PGPR) for sustainable agriculture. In: Bio-Based Nanoemulsions for Agri-Food Applications. Amsterdam, Netherlands: Elsevier; 2022. pp. 207-223

[115] Mohapatra S, Sarkar B, Samantaray DP, et al. Bioconversion of fish solid waste into PHB using *Bacillus subtilis* based submerged fermentation process. Environmental Technology. 2017;**38**:3201-3208

[116] Hong HA, Huang J-M, Khaneja R, et al. The safety of *Bacillus subtilis* and Bacillus indicus as food probiotics. Journal of Applied Microbiology. 2008;**105**:510-520

[117] Schallmey M, Singh A, Ward OP. Developments in the use of bacillus species for industrial production. Canadian Journal of Microbiology. 2004;**50**:1-17

[118] Brutscher LM, Borgmeier C, Garvey SM, et al. Preclinical safety assessment of *Bacillus subtilis* BS50 for probiotic and food applications. Microorganisms. 2022;**10**:1038

[119] EFSA Panel on Additives and Products or Substances used in Animal Feed (FEEDAP), Bampidis V, Azimonti G, et al. Safety and efficacy of a feed additive consisting of *Bacillus subtilis* strains CNCM I-4606, CNCM I-5043 and CNCM I-4607 and Lactococcus lactis CNCM I-4609 for all animal species (Nolivade). EFSA Journal. 2021;**19**:e06907

[120] Aquilina G, Bories G, Brantom P, et al. Scientific opinion on the safety and efficacy of *Bacillus subtilis* PB6 (*Bacillus*

subtilis) as a feed additive for chickens for fattening. EFSA Journal. 2009;7:1-14

[121] EFSA panel on additives and products or substances used in animal feed (FEEDAP). Scientific opinion on the safety and efficacy of *Bacillus subtilis* PB6 (*Bacillus subtilis*) as a feed additive for laying hens and minor poultry species for laying. EFSA Journal. 2015;**13**:3970

[122] Environmental Protection Agency, *Bacillus subtilis* Strain AFS032321; Exemption from the Requirement of a Tolerance. Federal Register; 2022. Available from: https://www.federalregister.gov/documents/2022/04/08/2022-07561/bacillus-subtilis-strain-afs032321-exemption-from-the-requirement-of-a-tolerance [Accessed: February 28, 2025]

[123] Ouoba LII, Thorsen L, Varnam AH. Enterotoxins and emetic toxins production by Bacillus cereus and other species of bacillus isolated from Soumbala and Bikalga, African alkaline fermented food condiments. International Journal of Food Microbiology. 2008;**124**:224-230

[124] Zielińska D, Sionek B, Kołożyn-Krajewska D. Chapter 6 - Safety of probiotics. In: Holban AM, Grumezescu AM, editors. Diet, Microbiome and Health. Cambridge, Massachusetts: Academic Press; 2018. pp. 131-161

[125] Haranahalli Nataraj B, Behare PV, Yadav H, et al. Emerging pre-clinical safety assessments for potential probiotic strains: A review. Critical Reviews in Food Science and Nutrition. 2024;**64**:8155-8183

[126] Merenstein D, Pot B, Leyer G, et al. Emerging issues in probiotic safety: 2023 perspectives. Gut Microbes. 2023;**15**:2185034

Section 2

B. subtilis Probiotic Power

Chapter 2

B. subtilis Probiotics for Humans, Animals and Plants: Mechanisms, Applications and Prospects

Dilan Ergün, Göksu Tartar and Ayten Yazgan-Karataş

Abstract

Bacillus bacteria have increasingly attracted research interest due to their promising probiotic properties, including strong antimicrobial, antidiarrheal, and immunostimulatory effects. They are able to stimulate the growth of natural flora, prevent intestinal inflammation, and demonstrate excellent stability even under adverse conditions. This chapter explores the probiotic applications of *Bacillus subtilis* strains in humans, animals, and plants. First, the chapter reviews the probiotic mechanisms of *B. subtilis* and the current state of research in this area. The potential applications of recombinant *B. subtilis* probiotics are also covered, along with results from preclinical studies and the future role of *B. subtilis* probiotic therapy in clinical settings. This chapter aims to survey the current landscape of *B. subtilis* probiotic research and hypothesize about its potential future impact.

Keywords: *B. subtilis*, probiotics, recombinant probiotics, biotherapy, live therapeutics

1. Introduction

The worldwide use of probiotics has increased due to their positive effects on the human microbiota and health [1]. Probiotics, as defined by the International Scientific Association for Probiotics and Prebiotics (ISAPP) panel in 2013, are live microorganisms that provide health benefits to the host when administered in sufficient quantities [2]. Most human dairy products contain probiotic bacteria, and the global market for probiotic supplements is growing significantly. *Lactobacillus* and *Bifidobacterium* are the most commonly used and commercialized genera [3, 4]. However, the genus *Lactobacillus* is microaerophilic, whereas the genus *Bifidobacterium* is strictly anaerobic. Furthermore, these genera are slow-growing and sensitive to temperature and gastric juices, leading to challenges in production, storage, and delivery processes [5]. Among these genera, the species *Bacillus subtilis* probiotics provide multifaceted advantages over conventional probiotics in several areas due to their advanced properties, including shelf stability, resistance to extreme environmental conditions, and safe interactions with humans, animals, and plants [6]. Moreover, *B. subtilis* has several distinctive characteristics, such as versatility in nutrient use for growth, spore formation, a high growth rate, growth in both aerobic and anaerobic environments, and high enzyme and antimicrobial production, making it an attractive bacterium for probiotic research [7].

Bacillus species have been utilized as probiotics for at least 60 years, with the 1958 registration of the Italian product Enterogermina as a medicinal supplement [8]. Of the *Bacillus* species, endospore-forming soil-dwelling *B. subtilis* is the most ubiquitous bacterium in diverse ecological settings ranging from terrestrial to aquatic environments [9]. This organism's genetics and physiology have been extensively researched, and the understanding of its genetic background and physiology is second only to that of *Escherichia coli* [10, 11]. Recent probiotic studies of *B. subtilis* have made significant advances in clarifying the spectrum of activity that makes this bacterium one of the most appealing probiotics [5]. *B. subtilis* strains have been studied as probiotics for their antibacterial, antifungal, antiviral, antidiarrheal, and immunostimulatory effects, as well as for their potential to compete with pathogens for survival, inhibit intestinal inflammation, and stimulate the growth of normal intestinal flora [12–17]. This chapter discusses the applications of *B. subtilis* probiotics in humans, animals, and plants. First, the chapter reviews the probiotic mechanisms of *B. subtilis* and the current state of research in this area. The potential applications of recombinant *B. subtilis* probiotics are also be covered, along with results from preclinical studies and the future role of *B. subtilis* probiotic therapy in clinical settings.

2. Mechanisms of action of *B. subtilis* probiotics

B. subtilis' probiotic effects on the host can be attributed to a variety of mechanisms, including antimicrobial effect, antidiarrheal effect, immunostimulatory effect, competitive exclusion of pathogens, prevention of intestinal inflammation, and stimulation of growth of intestinal normal flora [18].

2.1 Synthesis of antimicrobial agents

Both industry and healthcare have made extensive use of *Bacillus* spp. due to their ability to produce a wide range of biologically active metabolites, particularly antimicrobials [19]. Pathogenic infections are a leading cause of morbidity and mortality worldwide, and while synthetic antibiotics are used to control pathogenic overgrowth, their indiscriminate use leads to the emergence of multidrug-resistant pathogenic bacteria. *B. subtilis*, one of the most prominent species, has shown promise in this area by serving as a viable therapeutic antimicrobial, as it synthesizes 66 antibiotics and allocates 4–5% of its genome to antibiotic biosynthesis [1, 7, 20]. The antibiotics synthesized by *B. subtilis* have diverse structures and antimicrobial properties. Specifically, *B. subtilis* synthesizes antimicrobial agents that disrupt cell walls and plasma membranes and interfere with intracellular processes [19]. Bacilysin exerts its effect by targeting the cell walls of *Candida albicans* and foodborne pathogens such as *Escherichia coli*, *Salmonella enterica* and *Bacillus cereus* [21, 22]. *B. subtilis* biosynthesizes lipopeptide antibiotics such as surfactin and fengicyn, which exert their antimicrobial activity against harmful microorganisms such as plant pathogens such as *Rhizopus stolonifer* through their interaction mechanisms with phospholipid bilayer membranes [23, 24]. Some agents inhibit pathogens by disrupting intracellular processes without disrupting cell walls and plasma membranes; for example, sublancin, a glycosylated peptide produced by *B. subtilis* 168, shows antibacterial activity against methicillin-resistant *Staphylococcus aureus* by disrupting the central dogma [25, 26]. In this regard, *B. subtilis* probiotics are promising antibiotic substitutes with remarkable antimicrobial properties, highlighting their potential as a novel strategy to overcome microbial infections [27]. For example, supplementation with *B. subtilis* PB6 in *E. coli*-infected broilers reduced the mortality rate from 14% to 8%, while antibiotic administration reduced it to 6% [28]. Similarly, compared to negative controls, supplementation with *B. subtilis* DSM 32315 and Nasarin reduced mortality by 6.5% and 9.1%, respectively [29]. *B. subtilis* has also been shown to reduce *Salmonella typhimurium* infection in cell culture studies, in addition to mucosa-associated lymphoid tissue (MALT) healing [30].

2.2 Immunostimulatory effect

B. subtilis stimulates both specific and non-specific immunity, thereby improving protection against pathogens. *Bacillus* spores have been shown to stimulate the immune system by oral administration in numerous studies in humans and animal models. *B. subtilis* spores induce specific humoral and cell-mediated immune responses. The development of both innate and adaptive immune responses in the host is significantly influenced by the interaction between *B. subtilis* spores and macrophages [5]. Studies on macrophages and *B. subtilis* spore co-cultures showed that *B. subtilis* significantly increased the secretion of pro-inflammatory cytokines, including tumor necrosis factor-alpha (TNF-α), interferon-gamma (IFN-γ), interleukin-1 beta (IL-1β), IL-6, IL-8 and IL-12 [31–33]. Lefevre et al. [34] demonstrated that supplementation of elderly humans with *B. subtilis* CU1 significantly increased fecal and salivary secretory IgA concentrations compared to placebo. Administration of *B. subtilis* MBTU PBBM1 spores to mouse models resulted in T lymphocyte proliferation and accumulation of IgG and IgA antibodies, indicating the potential of *B. subtilis* MBTU PBBM1 spores to enhance both humoral and cellular immunity in mice [35]. Bai et al. [36] showed that administration of *B. subtilis* fmbJ to broilers significantly increased serum IgG and IgA levels. In addition, a study by Li et al. [37] in growing-finishing pigs showed that *B. subtilis* increased serum IgG levels, suggesting that supplementation with *B. subtilis* significantly stimulates the immune response. A study in a rabbit model showed that the combination of *Bacteroides fragilis* and *B. subtilis* had a positive effect on the development of gut-associated lymphoid tissue (GALT) and the diversification of the pre-immune antibody repertoire. Furthermore, two stress responses controlled by Spo0A, including sporulation and TapA (formerly YqxM) secretion, were found to be necessary for GALT development in *B. subtilis* [38].

2.3 Maintenance of intestinal homeostasis

Probiotic *B. subtilis* strains have shown promising results in supporting gastrointestinal health and exhibiting anti-inflammatory properties [5, 6]. Patch et al. [39] found that *B. subtilis* supplementation significantly improved symptoms of constipation, indigestion and dyspepsia compared to the placebo control group. Further research has shown that stool quality was significantly improved following *B. subtilis* supplementation, while stool frequency per day and abdominal noises were significantly reduced [40, 41]. In addition, anti-inflammatory immune cell populations increased in response to *ex vivo* lipopolysaccharide stimulation of peripheral blood mononuclear cells [42]. Studies in piglets and growing-finishing pigs showed that *B. subtilis* supplementation improved the efficiency of digestion and metabolism of nutrients and had antioxidant effects. *B. subtilis* was shown to have a positive effect on intestinal histomorphology and its supplementation could promote a more favorable mucosal structure and larger absorptive areas of the luminal villi, thus promoting better intestinal development [37, 43, 44]. This finding suggested the reason for the improved digestive efficiency [37]. It was also reported that administration of *B. subtilis* to pigs increased serum superoxide dismutase levels, and after administration of *B. subtilis* fmbJ, reactive oxygen species (ROS) levels in liver mitochondria of broilers were significantly decreased, and the expression of antioxidant enzyme genes including nuclear factor erythroid 2-related factor 2 (Nrf2), haem oxygenase 1 (HO-1), superoxide dismutase (SOD), and glutathione peroxidase (GPx) were improved. Irritable bowel syndrome and inflammatory bowel disease (IBD), which includes Crohn's disease and ulcerative colitis, have been shown to be associated with oxidative stress and may benefit from antioxidant effects that help maintain and restore intestinal function [45]. Studies in broilers showed that supplementation with *B. subtilis* increased goblet cells in the intestinal tract by 19% and reduced the severity of inflammatory cell infiltration in the jejunum [46, 47]. Research in mice showed that histological damage caused by IBD was reduced by the ingestion of *B. subtilis*, which upregulated the expression of tight junction proteins and suppressed cytokine expression to mitigate intestinal epithelial damage [48]. Furthermore, competence and sporulation factor (CSF) synthesized by *B. subtilis* was found to activate the p38 MAP kinase and protein kinase B (Akt) survival pathways in intestinal epithelial cells, preventing oxidant-induced intestinal epithelial cell injury and loss of barrier function after its OCTN2-mediated transport [49]. CSF also reduced intestinal inflammation and improved survival in mice with lethal colitis [50].

2.4 Maintenance of gut microbiota

B. subtilis administration has been shown to influence the gut microbiota profile by stimulating the growth of normal gut flora and by competitively eliminating pathogens [51]. Studies conducted in broilers showed that *B. subtilis* promoted the presence of beneficial bacteria in the gut such as *Enterococcus*, *Lactobacillus* spp., *Bifidobacterium* spp., *Firmicutes*, *Christensenellaceae*, *Caulobacteraceae*, *Ruminococcus*, *Lachnoclostridium*, and *Anaerostipes* while reducing *Vampirovibrio*, *Escherichia/Shigella*, *Parabacteroides*, *Clostridium*, *Coliforms*, *Campylobacter*, *Bacteroidetes*, and *E. coli* [52–58]. It has also been shown that adherence of *Salmonella enteritidis*, *Listeria monocytogenes*, and *Escherichia coli* pathogens to the HT-29 cell line was inhibited by *B. subtilis* P223 [16]. Furthermore, the *B. subtilis*-treated model organism *Bombyx mori* L. had a higher abundance of *Enterococcus* compared to the control group [59]. Studies in pigs and piglets exhibited that *B. subtilis* supplementation increased the numbers of *Lactobacilli*, *Leucobacter* and *Cupriavidus*, *Coprococcus*, and *Bifidobacterium*, as well as colonic *Succiniclasticum* cells the numbers of *Clostridium perfringens* and *E. coli* [43, 54, 60, 61]. Other studies have demonstrated that *B. subtilis* favors the intestinal colonization of some beneficial bacteria, including *Lactobacillus*, *Leucobacter*, *Bifidobacteria*, *Megasphaera*, *Coprococcus*, *Gemmatimonadete*, *Acidobacteria*, *Ruminococcaceae*_UCG-013 cc, and *Prevotella* [43, 62, 63]. Administration of *B. subtilis* has been shown to alter the microbial composition and optimize the structure of the gut microbiome, contributing to its beneficial effects as a probiotic [37, 43, 44, 63].

3. Applications of probiotic *B. subtilis*

3.1 For humans

Human studies have demonstrated the potential of *B. subtilis* probiotics to effectively treat various intestinal infections and diseases, including antibiotic-associated diarrhea, ulcerative colitis, acute intestinal infections, irritable bowel syndrome, and other infectious pathologies [5, 6]. In addition, probiotic *B. subtilis* has been shown to be effective in the treatment of immunodeficiency [64], Alzheimer's disease [65] and Parkinson's disease [66]. *B. subtilis*-derived probiotics have been shown to increase human longevity by slowing the progression of age-related diseases [67]. In addition, *B. subtilis* supplementation has been beneficial in reducing risk factors associated with cardiovascular disease by lowering cholesterol levels in the human bloodstream [68, 69]. Furthermore, the use of *B. subtilis* natto DG101 in conjunction with appropriate medication has become a promising and innovative intervention in the fight against the global diabetes epidemic [70].

B. subtilis has also shown promise as an adjunctive treatment for *Helicobacter pylori* eradication therapy and dysbacteriosis in neonates and children [5, 6]. Given its ability to favorably alter the gastrointestinal microflora, *B. subtilis* probiotics are being considered as a daily supplement to support overall gut and digestive health in individuals. Probiotic strains of *B. subtilis* have been shown to have beneficial effects on GI health, including improvements in constipation [39], GI quality of life [71], body composition [72–74], stool regularity [40, 41], GI discomfort [75], bloating and belching [76], and microbiome composition [41, 77]. Additional benefits have been observed in glucose metabolism [73], amino acid, purine and vitamin B metabolism [59], GI hormonal response [68, 78], anti-inflammatory activity [42], lipid metabolism [68, 72], endothelial function [68], bone density [79] and immune response [34].

In recent years, engineered probiotics have gained considerable attention as a live therapy to maintain healthy gut microbiota and treat microbial infections. *Lactobacillus rhamnosus* GG (LGG) is a widely studied probiotic for use in ulcerative colitis [80], diarrhea [81] and atopic dermatitis [82]. A major secreted protein, p75, enhances its probiotic activity by maintaining intestinal epithelial cell proliferation and survival by stimulating activation of Akt, suppressing cytokine-induced epithelial cell apoptosis, increasing cell proliferation and reducing tumor necrosis factor (TNF)-induced colonic epithelial damage [83, 84]. However, maintaining the viability of these probiotics during food processing and in the gut remains a challenge [85, 86]. A recent study anchored the p75 protein from *L. rhamnosus* GG to *B. subtilis* via CotG, demonstrating its antibacterial activity against the foodborne pathogen *Listeria monocytogenes* [27]. Researchers have also investigated *B. subtilis* probiotics as a vaccine delivery system. These spore probiotics enhance immune responses by presenting antigens in the gut [87]. For example, researchers have proposed *B. subtilis* spores expressing *H. pylori* urease B (UreB) protein on their surface as a promising oral vaccine against *H. pylori* infection. In experimental mouse models, oral administration of UreB-expressing recombinant *B. subtilis* spores resulted in a significant humoral immune response. Furthermore, oral administration of these engineered spores reduced *H. pylori* load in infected mice by 84% compared to the control group [88]. Several studies have highlighted the importance of surface display of antigens on *B. subtilis* probiotics, such as the C fragment of tetanus toxin (TTFC) [89], the tegument protein of *Clonorchis sinensis* [90] and the SARS-CoV-2 spike protein [91]. These studies have shown that oral administration of these engineered *B. subtilis* probiotics induces robust immune responses.

Researchers are exploring novel approaches to promote gut health, modify metabolic pathways and improve overall health through the development of recombinant *B. subtilis* probiotic candidates, paving the way for a new era in the treatment of infectious diseases and metabolic disorders. For example, a recent study evaluated the efficacy of a novel recombinant *B. subtilis* SP-64 strain expressing human alcohol dehydrogenase-4 (ADH4) in mice to treat diet-induced metabolic disorders such as obesity, fatty liver disease and type 2 diabetes [1]. Long-term ethanol production in the gastrointestinal (GI) system can damage the gut microbiota and cause organ dysfunction. It is necessary to reduce ethanol exposure to internal organs and increase ADH4 activity, which is necessary for alcohol metabolism [92]. In the study, increased rates of ethanol removal were achieved with the customized *B. subtilis*. Treatment with this customized probiotic significantly reduced weight gain in mice, promoted glucose utilization and prevented pancreatic damage from a high-fat diet [1]. A recent study investigated a lactate oxidase-expressing recombinant *B. subtilis* as a therapeutic probiotic candidate for metabolic disorders associated with elevated blood lactate levels [93]. Anaerobic glycolysis can lead to elevated lactate levels associated with diseases such as cancer, diabetes and mitochondrial dysfunction [94–96]. Traditional techniques for treating elevated lactate levels, such as small molecule inhibitors or enzyme replacement, have limited clinical efficacy [97–99]. In this study, lactate oxidase (LOX)-expressing recombinant *B. subtilis* probiotic candidates were orally administered to the mouse models to improve the rate of removal of elevated blood lactate levels and combat associated metabolic diseases. Oral administration of these LOX-expressing recombinant spore-based *B. subtilis* probiotics significantly reduced elevated blood lactate levels in the animal models without affecting the immune system, liver or gut microbiome [93].

3.2 For animals

Livestock production has expanded significantly to meet the needs of a growing global population, with antibiotics being used as growth promoters to improve feed conversion rates [100–102]. However, this has led to the development of antibiotic-resistant pathogenic bacteria that pose a threat to human health and the economy [103, 104]. The rise of antimicrobial resistance has reduced effective treatments, reduced animal productivity and increased the risk of infectious diseases [105]. The use of antibiotic growth promoters as feed additives has been prohibited in many countries due to regulatory pressure and consumer demand [106]. Alternatives such as probiotics, feed enzymes, prebiotic oligosaccharides, synbiotics, essential oils and immunostimulants have gained interest to maintain current animal production metrics [107]. As a promising probiotic alternative, *B. subtilis* strains have long been used as feed additives to promote animal growth and prevent disease [108]. Its ability to be produced in the form of endospores allows it to rapidly reactivate in the upper intestine to secrete proteases, facilitating the breakdown of complex carbohydrates in plant diets [109–111]. *B. subtilis* produces antimicrobial agents that fight intestinal pathogens and improve intestinal health and food absorption [19–24, 47, 51].

Animal feed production processes typically require high temperatures, and spore-producing bacteria are well suited to these conditions. In the production of functional animal feeds, the ability to sporulate, grow under both aerobic and anaerobic conditions, and survive inside and outside of humans and animals makes the *B. subtilis* strains one of the most versatile and attractive probiotic bacteria [7, 107]. Several studies have evaluated the effects of *B. subtilis* probiotics on broiler growth performance compared to antibiotics. Lee et al. [112] found that broilers supplemented with *B. subtilis* had higher body weights than those supplemented with 60 mg/kg salinomycin. Teo and Tan [28] showed that the administration of *B. subtilis* PB6 to *E. coli*-infected broilers improved the average daily gain from day 21 to 41 by 7.5% compared to the administration of a combination of 16.7 mg/kg bacitracin zinc and 3.3 mg/kg colistin sulfate. In addition, recombinant *B. subtilis* probiotics in Eimeria maxima-infected broilers significantly improved gut integrity, enhanced innate immunity, and improved growth performance in young chickens [113]. In addition, a study proposed *Clostridium perfringens* alpha toxoid expressing recombinant *B. subtilis* as a promising vaccine for the prevention of necrotic enteritis in poultry [114]. *B. subtilis* spore probiotics expressing a truncated Newcastle disease virus haemagglutinin-neuraminidase protein and a *B. subtilis* strain expressing the duck hepatitis A virus type 1 VP1 protein significantly induced strong systemic and mucosal immune responses in mice, highlighting the potential of *B. subtilis* probiotics as an immunization agent for poultry [115, 116]. The *B. subtilis* probiotic strain was also genetically modified to detoxify poultry feed by inserting the dioxin degradation system of *Sphingomonas wittichii*. It significantly reduced dioxin levels, demonstrating its potential as a feed additive to detoxify poultry diets and provide safe consumption for chickens [117].

Newborn piglets have a sterile gut that eventually develops their characteristic microbiome through interaction with the sow and surrounding environment. The periods immediately following birth and post-weaning represent the most vulnerable stages in a pig's lifecycle, where the elimination of antimicrobial substances from feed could impact mortality rates [118, 119]. A recombinant *B. subtilis* probiotic expressing antimicrobial peptide was developed to address these issues in swine production. Tests on the constructed recombinant probiotics *in vitro* exhibited antimicrobial activity against *E. coli*, *S. typhimurium*, *Haemophilus parasuis*, and *S. aureus*. Furthermore, administration of these engineered probiotics in weaned piglets significantly enhanced the growth and reduced the incidence of diarrhea from enteropathogenic *E. coli* challenge compared to non-supplemented piglets [120].

Porcine epidemic diarrhea virus (PEDV) is a serious pig disease causing high mortality from diarrhea in piglets [121–123]. Currently, available PEDV vaccines lack efficacy, resulting in inadequate treatment [124, 125]. As *B. subtilis* probiotics are known to improve immune regulation and promote gut health in pigs when administered orally [126], engineering *B. subtilis* probiotics to provide immunization against PEDV infection is a promising approach to overcome the current challenges in treating PEDV infection [127]. These probiotics could also be developed as feed additives with enhanced nutritional value. Previous work has shown that tryptophan-excreting *B. subtilis* probiotics can produce tryptophan *in situ* to supplement pig diets, offering the potential benefits of reducing environmental pollution from nitrogen sources and feed costs [128].

Live microbial feed additives, such as probiotics, may not only alter the rumen microbiota but also induce strong host immune responses [129, 130]. Higher feed efficiency and improved milk production have been demonstrated in cows fed *B. subtilis* natto fermentation products, suggesting that *B. subtilis* natto alters rumen fermentation patterns [129, 131]. *Haemonchus contortus* is an important gastrointestinal parasite that infects sheep, causing blood loss and anemia. *H. contortus* infection affects the gastrointestinal microbial population, inhibiting protein digestion and growth performance in infected animals [132, 133]. A recent study showed that HcGAPDH protein from *H. contortus* expressing a recombinant probiotic *B. subtilis* strain induced immune responses in sheep and reduced worm burden [134].

3.3 For plants

Biological products containing live bacterial cells and/or their metabolites have great potential as next-generation methods of crop protection. These technological advances now allow plant breeders to potentially avoid reliance on chemical pesticide and fungicide applications in some cases. *B. subtilis*, in particular, has shown promise as an effective biological control alternative to chemical control [135, 136]. *B. subtilis* is a common plant growth-promoting rhizobacterium (PGPR) that enhances plant development and yield. It protects the plant against stress through biofilm development, lipopeptide production, siderophore secretion and exopolysaccharide release. It acts as an effective denitrifying agent in the agroecosystem and maintains soil health through environmentally sustainable remediation approaches [137]. For example, the use of *B. subtilis* as a biofertilizer in fertigated Tarocco blood orange groves has been shown to improve fruit quality, soil fertility, growth and nutrient uptake, and to reduce the need for chemical fertilizers [138]. Field trials using *B. subtilis* CPA-8 have reduced *Monilinia* spp. plant infections, demonstrating its potential as an environmentally friendly alternative to fungicides [135]. The chitinase from *Bacillus pumilus* was expressed on *B. subtilis* spores and its biopesticidal activity was demonstrated against fungal pathogens such as *Rhizoctonia solani* and *Trichoderma harzianum*, which are major threats to maintaining sustainable agriculture, highlighting the potential of these novel biocontrol agents [139].

4. Clinical trials

Functional gastrointestinal disorders affect 25–40% of the world's population. They are chronic conditions with persistent symptoms, including functional bowel disorders, irritable bowel syndrome, constipation, diarrhea and bloating [39, 140]. Antibiotics are often ineffective or contraindicated for long-term use, whereas probiotics offer health benefits without resistance [141]. A clinical trial investigated the use of probiotic *B. subtilis* (BG01-4TM) in the treatment of functional gastrointestinal disorders and found that BG01-4TM relieved constipation symptoms, suggesting its potential in the treatment of GI dysfunction [39]. A study of 400 adult patients with moderate-to-severe diarrhea-predominant irritable bowel syndrome (IBS-D) found that *B. subtilis* containing Bio-Kult®, a multi-strain probiotic, reduced abdominal pain and improved bowel movements, suggesting potential benefits for IBS-D patients [142]. A clinical trial in 76 healthy subjects found that daily *B. subtilis* BS50 supplementation for 6 weeks improved bloating, belching and flatulence, suggesting a safe approach to gastrointestinal discomfort [76]. A study in 81 healthy adults aged 18–50 years evaluated the tolerability and safety of *B. subtilis* R0179. The study found no adverse effects on general well-being or gastrointestinal function. *B. subtilis* R0179 was well tolerated at doses ranging from 0.1 to 10×10^9 cfu/day [75].

In a recent study, two cases of type 2 diabetes were well controlled with *B. subtilis* natto DG101 probiotics. Probiotics helped control blood glucose and insulin levels in two cases of type 2 diabetes in obese patients. This study shows the potential of *B. subtilis* probiotics in managing type 2 diabetes and in maintaining health and managing disease [70].

5. Future prospects

Recently, *B. subtilis* as a probiotic has gained attention for its applications in skin care. A study in mice showed that a *B. subtilis*-supplemented Pluronic F-127 hydrogel could modulate the skin microbiome, revealing its potential in the treatment of skin dysbiosis-related diseases such as atopic dermatitis, acne, rosacea, and psoriasis [143]. Furthermore, topical application of *B. subtilis*-substituted polyvinyl alcohol (PVA) microparticles effectively reduced the healing time of open wounds in mice, indicating the potential of *B. subtilis* as an effective therapeutic agent for acute or chronic open wounds [144]. Despite its promising potential, there is a lack of scientifically validated clinical data on the efficacy and safety of probiotic *B. subtilis* formulations for the treatment of skin disorders, which could be urgently pursued as future research.

Psychobiotic strains influence central nervous system (CNS)-related functions and behaviors mediated by the gut-brain axis (GBA) through a number of different pathways [145]. There is growing interest among researchers in the field of microbial-based psychopharmaceuticals. An imbalance in the gut microbiota has been linked to a range of health problems, including inflammatory bowel disease, obesity, type 2 diabetes, and even mental health conditions such as autism, Alzheimer's disease (AD), depression and anxiety [146]. In recent years, preclinical and some clinical studies of psychobiotics have yielded encouraging results in the treatment of neurodegenerative and depressive disorders [65, 147]. Bacteria of the genera *Lactobacillus* and *Bifidobacterium* have been most extensively studied for their psychobiotic effects [146, 147]. Conversely, recent studies have shown that *B. subtilis* strains also have promising psychobiotic properties. For example, studies using chickens as a model organism have shown that *B. subtilis* has beneficial effects on growth performance, intestinal microstructure and digestive enzymes, synthesis and release of antimicrobial and antibiotic compounds, immunity and neurotransmitter activities, including serotonin, and animal behavior following various stressors. In addition, *B. subtilis* has the ability to overproduce L-tryptophan, which subsequently increases 5-HT in the hypothalamus, acting as an antidepressant and anti-anxiety agent, relieving nervous tension in mice and reducing aggressive behavior in laying hens [148]. Besides serotonin, *B. subtilis* has the ability to produce gamma-aminobutyric acid (GABA) [149, 150]. GABA is one of the most important inhibitors in the brain, regulating many physiological and psychological processes. Its dysfunction has been implicated in anxiety and depression. It also plays an important role in the prevention of neurological diseases, cancer, type 1 diabetes and immune disorders [151]. Nitric oxide (NO), another neurotransmitter involved in several GI functions, including maintaining vascular tone, modulating immune responses, transmitting nerve impulses, and facilitating GI motility by relaxing intestinal muscles, could be produced by *B. subtilis* [152]. Alzheimer's disease (AD) is a major cause of dementia among diseases of the nervous system. The exact etiology of Alzheimer's disease remains incompletely understood. There is no definitive and effective treatment for the disease. *B. subtilis* NCIB 3610 has been extensively studied for its ability to form well-structured, three-dimensional biofilms *in vitro*, which is one of the many potential pathways by which it exerts a probiotic effect [153]. It has been shown to delay the onset of age-related neurodegenerative and cognitive deficits in a *Caenorhabditis elegans* model of AD [65]. The anti-AD effects of *B. subtilis* are directly related to the ability of the probiotic to synthesize a quorum-sensing peptide—Competence Sporulation Factor (CSF)—and to gut-associated biofilm development. Alpha-synuclein (αSyn), a highly soluble unfolded protein, has been implicated in Alzheimer's disease and Parkinson's disease. A reduction in DA levels in αSyn has been observed in post-mortem AD brains, which is associated with cognitive decline. Another *B. subtilis* PXN21 has been observed to inhibit, delay and even reverse αSyn aggregation in young and old *C. elegans* models by altering the sphingolipid metabolic pathway. Despite these promising results, scientifically validated research into their psychobiotic effects has been limited. Their effects may vary depending on factors such as strain type, dosage and individual differences. Comprehensive molecular mechanism studies, animal experiments and clinical trials are therefore essential to refine their use [65, 154, 155].

The potential therapeutic efficacy of *B. subtilis* against coronavirus disease (COVID-19) has recently been elucidated [156]. By modulating the immune system, *B. subtilis* appears to help prevent excessive inflammation and thus improve patient outcomes. Preliminary evidence suggests that this bacterium may have an inhibitory effect on viral replication. This observation warrants further investigation, particularly given the lack of clarity regarding its specific activity against the severe acute respiratory syndrome coronavirus 2 (SARS-CoV-2) virus. *B. subtilis* is still being tested as a treatment for patients with COVID-19 [156] and further studies are needed to confirm its potential and understand how it works.

Recent advances in "omics" technologies, including genomics, transcriptomics, proteomics and metabolomics, have significantly improved our understanding of *B. subtilis* at the molecular level. By integrating omic approaches with systems biology studies, researchers have gained insight into the networks and pathways that control the physiology of this model bacterium [157]. Advances in synthetic biology and genome editing techniques such as CRISPR-Cas9 have led to the development of engineered probiotics for various health problems. These probiotics can be used to treat inflammatory bowel disease, cancer and neurological disorders. *B. subtilis*, known for its non-pathogenicity, excellent protein secretion ability, adaptive metabolism and resistance, makes it an ideal candidate for metabolic engineering and synthetic biology to produce live therapeutics for disease treatment [6, 158]. An intriguing example of such applications is the genetically engineered probiotic *Bacillus subtilis* ZB183, which is Food and Drug Administration (FDA)-compliant and has been developed with the ability to reduce alcohol hangover. This product has been marketed by ZBiotics since 2019 [159, 160]. In addition, in 2024, ZBiotics commercialized another engineered probiotic bacterium, ZB423™, to convert sugar into fiber continuously throughout the day. This unique probiotic produces levansucrase, an enzyme that splits sugar into glucose and fructose, and redirects the fructose to form a rare fiber called levan. This enzyme is delivered directly to the gut, maximizing the benefits and delivering the fiber in a way that is preferred by the microbiome [161, 162]. These two recombinant commercial examples represent a significant advance demonstrating the success and safety of engineered *B. subtilis* probiotics, the number of which is expected to increase rapidly in the near future.

6. Conclusions

The *Bacillus* genus of bacteria has recently become the subject of considerable research interest, due to the significant potential health benefits they offer to humans, animals and plants. For humans, *B. subtilis* offers a wide range of health-promoting properties, including improved digestion, stimulation of the growth of natural microflora, circulatory blood homeostasis, stimulation of the immune system, prevention of intestinal inflammation, and potential protection against pathogenic invaders. Clinical trials have demonstrated the safety and efficacy of *B. subtilis* as a dietary supplement for the treatment of diseases affecting the gastrointestinal (GI) tract and type-II diabetes. In addition, preclinical studies have also yielded promising results for the management of cardiovascular diseases, inflammatory disorders, dermatological diseases, neurodegenerative and depressive conditions, and even SARS-CoV-2 infection.

B. subtilis is being used more in livestock farming because it improves feed efficiency and eliminates the need for antibiotics. This is achieved by improving nutrient digestibility, reducing pathogen load, strengthening mucosal physiology and improving gut immunity and microbiota diversity in various livestock species. Together with these beneficial effects, the capacity of *B. subtilis* to form spores at high temperatures and to survive in low pH environments renders it a robust strain that can be developed into an in-feed probiotic supplement.

The *B. subtilis* species is of great importance in maintaining plant health, promoting plant growth and fighting against pathogens. *B. subtilis* has been demonstrated to be highly effective in combating pathogens, enhancing nutrient availability and enhancing stress tolerance in plants. This highlights its significant potential in shaping the trajectory of sustainable agriculture.

The advent of synthetic biology with the advancement of genome editing techniques such as CRISPR-Cas9 has engendered promising prospects for the customization of *B. subtilis* strains. As a proficient chassis cell, these organisms can be modified to alter their intrinsic properties, thereby facilitating the development of novel solutions for the treatment of a spectrum of human, animal and plant diseases. Given its status as a commensal organism present in humans, animals and plants, its exceptional resilience even in adverse conditions and its designation as a Generally Recognized as Safe (GRAS) organism, engineered *B. subtilis* probiotics are poised to assume an even more pivotal role in sustainable practices and innovative solutions to the challenges of human, animal and plant health in the near future.

Author details

Dilan Ergün[1,2], Göksu Tartar[1,2] and Ayten Yazgan-Karataş[1,2]*

1 Department of Molecular Biology and Genetics, Faculty of Science and Letters, Istanbul Technical University, Istanbul, Turkiye

2 Dr. Orhan Ocalgiray Molecular Biology Biotechnology and Genetics Research Center, Istanbul Technical University, Istanbul, Turkiye

*Address all correspondence to: karatasay@itu.edu.tr

References

[1] Singh RP, Shadan A, Ma Y. Biotechnological applications of probiotics: A multifarious weapon to disease and metabolic abnormality. Probiotics and Antimicrobial Proteins. 2022;**14**(6):1184. DOI: 10.1007/S12602-022-09992-8

[2] Hill C, Guarner F, Reid G, Gibson GR, Merenstein DJ, Pot B, et al. Expert consensus document. The International Scientific Association for Probiotics and Prebiotics consensus statement on the scope and appropriate use of the term probiotic. Nature Reviews Gastroenterology & Hepatology. 2014;**11**(8):506-514. DOI: 10.1038/NRGASTRO.2014.66

[3] Chen J, Chen X, Ho CL. Recent development of probiotic bifidobacteria for treating human diseases. Frontiers in Bioengineering and Biotechnology. 2021;**9**:770248. DOI: 10.3389/FBIOE.2021.770248/

[4] Venkatesh GP, Kuruvalli G, Syed K, Reddy VD. An updated review on probiotic production and applications. Gastroenterology Insights. 2024;**1**:221-236. DOI: 10.3390/GASTROENT15010016

[5] Suva M, Sureja V, Kheni D. Novel insight on probiotic *B. subtilis*: Mechanism of action and clinical applications. Journal of Current Research in Scientific Medicine. 2016;**2**(2):65. DOI: 10.4103/2455-3069.198381

[6] Williams N, Weir TL. Spore-based probiotic *B. subtilis*: Current applications in humans and future. Perspectives. 2024;**10**(2):78. DOI: 10.3390/FERMENTATION10020078

[7] Olmos J, Paniagua-Michel J. *B. subtilis* a potential probiotic bacterium to formulate functional feeds for aquaculture. Journal of Microbial & Biochemical Technology. 2014;**06**(07):361-365. DOI: 10.4172/1948-5948.1000169

[8] Cutting SM. *Bacillus* probiotics. Food Microbiology. 2011;**28**(2):214-220. DOI: 10.1016/J.FM.2010.03.007

[9] Earl AM, Losick R, Kolter R. Ecology and genomics of *B. subtilis*. Trends in Microbiology. 2008;**16**(6):269-275. DOI: 10.1016/J.TIM.2008.03.004

[10] Kunst F, Ogasawara N, Moszer I, Albertini AM, Alloni G, Azevedo V, et al. The complete genome sequence of the gram-positive bacterium *B. subtilis*. Nature. 1997;**390**(6657):249-256. DOI: 10.1038/36786

[11] Driks A. Proteins of the spore core and coat. In: Sonenshein H, Losi, editorsck. *B. subtilis* and Its Closest Relatives. Washington, D.C: ASM Press; 2014. pp. 527-535. DOI: 10.1128/9781555817992.ch36

[12] Ritter A, Correa A, Veras F, Brandelli A. Characterization of *B. subtilis* available as probiotic. Journal of Microbiology Research. 2018;**8**(2):23-32. DOI: 10.5923/j.microbiology.20180802.01

[13] Starosila D, Rybalko S, Varbanetz L, Ivanskaya N, Sorokulova I. Anti-influenza activity of a *B. subtilis* probiotic strain. Antimicrobial Agents and Chemotherapy. 2017;**61**(7):e00539-17. DOI: 10.1128/AAC.00539-17

[14] Urdaci MC, Lefevre M, Lafforgue G, Cartier C, Rodriguez B, Fioramonti J. Antidiarrheal action of *B. subtilis* CU1 CNCM I-2745 and *L. plantarum* CNCM I-4547 in Mice. Frontiers in Microbiology. 2018;**9**:1537. DOI: 10.3389/FMICB.2018.01537

[15] Huang JM, la Ragione RM, Nunez A, Cutting SM. Immunostimulatory activity of *Bacillus* spores. FEMS Immunology and Medical Microbiology. 2008;**53**(2):195-203. DOI: 10.1111/J.1574-695X.2008.00415.X

[16] Jeon HL, Lee NK, Yang SJ, Kim WS, Paik HD. Probiotic characterization of *B. subtilis* P223 isolated from kimchi. Food Science and Biotechnology. 2017;**26**(6):1641-1648. DOI: 10.1007/S10068-017-0148-5

[17] Rhayat L, Maresca M, Nicoletti C, Perrier J, Brinch KS, Christian S, et al. Effect of *B. subtilis* strains on intestinal barrier function and inflammatory response. Frontiers in Immunology. 2019;**10**:564. DOI: 10.3389/FIMMU.2019.00564

[18] Leser TD, Knarreborg A, Worm J. Germination and outgrowth of *B. subtilis* and *B. licheniformis* spores in the gastrointestinal tract of pigs. Journal of Applied Microbiology. 2008;**104**(4):1025-1033. DOI: 10.1111/J.1365-2672.2007.03633.X

[19] Tran C, Cock IE, Chen X, Feng Y. Antimicrobial *Bacillus*: Metabolites and their mode of action. Antibiotics. 2022;**11**(1):88. DOI: 10.3390/ANTIBIOTICS11010088/S1

[20] Sorokulova I. Modern status and perspectives of *Bacillus* bacteria as probiotics. Journal of Probiotics and Health. 2013;**1**(4):e106. DOI: 10.4172/2329-8901.1000e106

[21] Wang T, Liu X-h, Wu M-b, Ge S. Molecular insights into the antifungal mechanism of bacilysin. Journal of Molecular Modeling. 2018;**24**(5):112. DOI: 10.1007/S00894-018-3645-4

[22] Nannan C, Vu HQ, Gillis A, Caulier S, Nguyen TTT, Mahillon J. Bacilysin within the *B. subtilis* group: Gene prevalence versus antagonistic activity against Gram-negative foodborne pathogens. Journal of Biotechnology. 2021;**327**:28-35. DOI: 10.1016/J.JBIOTEC.2020.12.017

[23] Tao Y, Bie X-m, Lv F-x, Zhao H-z, Lu Z-x. Antifungal activity and mechanism of fengycin in the presence and absence of commercial surfactin against *Rhizopus stolonifer*. Journal of Microbiology. 2011;**49**(1):146-150. DOI: 10.1007/S12275-011-0171-9

[24] Zhao H, Shao D, Jiang C, Shi J, Li Q, Huang Q, et al. Biological activity of lipopeptides from *Bacillus*. Applied Microbiology and Biotechnology. 2017;**101**(15):5951-5960. DOI: 10.1007/S00253-017-8396-0

[25] Wang S, Wang Q, Zeng X, Ye Q, Huang S, Yu H, et al. Use of the antimicrobial peptide sublancin with combined antibacterial and immunomodulatory activities to protect against methicillin-resistant *S. aureus* infection in mice. Journal of Agricultural and Food Chemistry. 2017;**65**(39):8595-8605. DOI: 10.1021/ACS.JAFC.7B02592

[26] Wu C, Biswas S, Garcia De Gonzalo CV, van der Donk WA. Investigations into the mechanism of action of sublancin. ACS Infectious Diseases. 2019;**5**(3):454-459. DOI: 10.1021/ACSINFECDIS.8B00320/

[27] Kang SJ, Jun JS, Moon JA, Hong KW. Surface display of p75, a *L. rhamnosus* GG derived protein, on *B. subtilis* spores and its antibacterial activity against *L. monocytogenes*. AMB Express. 2020;**10**(1):1-9. DOI: 10.1186/S13568-020-01073-9

[28] Teo AYL, Tan HM. Effect of *B. subtilis* PB6 (CloSTAT) on broilers infected with a pathogenic strain of *E. coli*. Journal of Applied Poultry Research.

2006;**15**(2):229-235. DOI: 10.1093/JAPR/15.2.229

[29] Whelan RA, Doranalli K, Rinttilä T, Vienola K, Jurgens G, Apajalahti J. The impact of *B. subtilis* DSM 32315 on the pathology, performance, and intestinal microbiome of broiler chickens in a necrotic enteritis challenge. Poultry Science. 2019;**98**(9):3450-3463. DOI: 10.3382/PS/PEY500

[30] Ostovan R, Pourmontaseri M, Hosseinzadeh S, Shekarforoush SS. Interaction between the probiotic *B. subtilis* and *S. typhimurium* in Caco-2 cell culture. Iranian Journal of Microbiology. 2021;**13**(1):91. DOI: 10.18502/IJM.V13I1.5497

[31] Huang Q, Xu X, Mao Y-l, Huang Y, Rajput IR, Li W-f. Effects of *B. subtilis* B10 spores on viability and biological functions of murine macrophages. Animal Science Journal. 2013;**84**(3):247-252. DOI: 10.1111/J.1740-0929.2012.01064.X

[32] Huang Q, Li YL, Xu X, Huang Y, Cui ZY, Yu DY, et al. Modulatory effects of *B. subtilis* BS02 on viability and immune responses of RAW 264.7 murine macrophages. Journal of Animal and Veterinary Advances. 2012;**11**(11):1934-1938

[33] Xu X, Huang Q, Mao Y, Cui Z, Li Y, Huang Y, et al. Immunomodulatory effects of *B. subtilis* (natto) B4 spores on murine macrophages. Microbiology and Immunology. 2012;**56**(12):817-824. DOI: 10.1111/J.1348-0421.2012.00508.X

[34] Lefevre M, Racedo SM, Ripert G, Housez B, Cazaubiel M, Maudet C, et al. Probiotic strain *B. subtilis* CU1 stimulates immune system of elderly during common infectious disease period: A randomized, double-blind placebo-controlled study. Immunity & Ageing. 2015;**12**(1):1-11. DOI: 10.1186/S12979-015-0051-Y/

[35] Keerthi T. Immunomodulatory effect of probiotic strain *B. subtilis* MBTU PBBM1 spores in Balb/c Mice. International Journal of Engineering and Technical Research. 2014;**2**:258

[36] Bai K, Huang Q, Zhang J, He J, Zhang L, Wang T. Supplemental effects of probiotic *B. subtilis* fmbJ on growth performance, antioxidant capacity, and meat quality of broiler chickens. Poultry Science. 2017;**96**(1):74-82. DOI: 10.3382/PS/PEW246

[37] Li R, Liu J, Liu Y, Cao L, Qiu W, Qin M. Probiotic effects of *B. subtilis* on growth performance and intestinal microecological balance of growing-to-finishing pigs. Journal of Food Biochemistry. 2023;**1**:7150917. DOI: 10.1155/2023/7150917

[38] Rhee KJ, Sethupathi P, Driks A, Lanning DK, Knight KL. Role of commensal bacteria in development of gut-associated lymphoid tissues and preimmune antibody repertoire. The Journal of Immunology;**172**(2):1118-1124. DOI: 10.4049/jimmunol.172.2.1118

[39] Patch C, Pearce AJ, Cheng M, Boyapati R, Brenna JT. *B. subtilis* (BG01-4TM) improves self-reported symptoms for constipation, indigestion, and dyspepsia: A phase 1/2A randomized controlled trial. Nutrients. 2023;**15**(21):4490. DOI: 10.3390/NU15214490

[40] Cuentas AM, Deaton J, Davidson J, Ardita C. The effect of *B. subtilis* DE111 on the daily bowel movement profile for people with occasional gastrointestinal irregularity. Journal of Probiotics and Health. 2017;**5**(4):1000189. DOI: 10.4172/2329-8901.1000189

[41] Hatanaka M, Yamamoto K, Suzuki N, Iio S, Takara T, Morita H, et al. Effect of *B. subtilis* C-3102 on loose stools in healthy volunteers. Beneficial Microbes. 2018;**9**(3):357-366. DOI: 10.3920/BM2017.0103

[42] Freedman KE, Hill JL, Wei Y, Vazquez AR, Grubb DS, Trotter RE, et al. Examining the gastrointestinal and immunomodulatory effects of the novel probiotic *B. subtilis* DE111. International Journal of Molecular Sciences. 2021;**22**(5):2453. DOI: 10.3390/IJMS22052453

[43] Ding H, Zhao X, Ma C, Gao Q, Yin Y, Kong X, et al. Dietary supplementation with *B. subtilis* DSM 32315 alters the intestinal microbiota and metabolites in weaned piglets. Journal of Applied Microbiology. 2021;**130**(1):217-232. DOI: 10.1111/jam.14767

[44] Tang W, Qian Y, Yu B, Zhang T, Gao J, He J, et al. Effects of *B. subtilis* DSM32315 supplementation and dietary crude protein level on performance, gut barrier function and microbiota profile in weaned piglets. Journal of Animal Science. 2019;**97**(5):2125-2138. DOI: 10.1093/jas/skz090

[45] Khan I, Samson SE, Grover AK. Antioxidant supplements and gastrointestinal diseases: A critical appraisal. Medical Principles and Practice. 2017;**26**(3):201. DOI: 10.1159/000468988

[46] Lourenco M, Kuritza L, Westphal P, Muniz E, Pickler L, Santin E. Effects of *B. subtilis* in the dynamics of infiltration of immunological cells in the intestinal mucosa of chickens challenged with *S. minnesota*. International Journal of Poultry Science. 2012;**11**:630-634. DOI: 10.3923/ijps.2012.630.634

[47] Koli D, Kadam M, Gole M, Patil A, Hajare S, Yeskal A, et al. Efficacy of *B. subtilis* (Gallipro) supplementation in *C. perfringens* challenged necrotic enteritis of broiler chicken. Indian Journal of Animal Research. 2018;**52**(4):619-622. DOI: 10.18805/IJAR.B-3253

[48] Gong Y, Li H, Li Y. Effects of *B. subtilis* on epithelial tight junctions of mice with inflammatory bowel disease. Journal of Interferon & Cytokine Research: The Official Journal of the International Society for Interferon and Cytokine Research. 2016;**36**(2):75-85. DOI: 10.1089/JIR.2015.0030

[49] Fujiya M, Musch MW, Nakagawa Y, Hu S, Alverdy J, Kohgo Y, et al. The *B. subtilis* quorum-sensing molecule CSF contributes to intestinal homeostasis via OCTN2, a host cell membrane transporter. Cell Host & Microbe. 2007;**1**(4):299-308. DOI: 10.1016/J.CHOM.2007.05.004

[50] Okamoto K, Fujiya M, Nata T, Ueno N, Inaba Y, Ishikawa C, et al. Competence and sporulation factor derived from *B. subtilis* improves epithelial cell injury in intestinal inflammation via immunomodulation and cytoprotection. International Journal of Colorectal Disease. 2012;**27**(8):1039-1046. DOI: 10.1007/S00384-012-1416-8

[51] Ricke SC, Saengkerdsub S. *Bacillus* probiotics and biologicals for improving animal and human health: Current applications and future prospects. In: Rai, Bai, editos. Beneficial Microbes in Fermented and Functional Foods. Boca Raton: CRC Press; 2014. pp. 341-360. DOI: 10.1201/b17912

[52] Ma Y, Wang W, Zhang H, Wang J, Zhang W, Gao J, et al. Supplemental *B. subtilis* DSM 32315 manipulates intestinal structure and microbial composition in broiler chickens. Scientific Reports. 2018;**8**(1):1-13. DOI: 10.1038/s41598-018-33762-8

[53] Wu BQ, Zhang T, Guo LQ, Lin JF. Effects of *B. subtilis* KD1 on broiler intestinal flora. Poultry Science. 2011;**90**(11):2493-2499. DOI: 10.3382/PS.2011-01529

[54] Guo X, Li D, Lu W, Piao X, Chen X. Screening of *Bacillus* strains as potential probiotics and subsequent confirmation of the in vivo effectiveness of *B. subtilis* MA139 in pigs. Antonie van Leeuwenhoek International Journal of General and Molecular Microbiology. 2006;**90**(2):139-146. DOI: 10.1007/s10482-006-9067-9

[55] Ciurescu G, Dumitru M, Gheorghe A, Untea AE, Drăghici R. Effect of *B. subtilis* on growth performance, bone mineralization, and bacterial population of broilers fed with different protein sources. Poultry Science. 2020;**99**(11):5960-5971. DOI: 10.1016/J.PSJ.2020.08.075

[56] Forte C, Acuti G, Manuali E, Casagrande Proietti P, Pavone S, Trabalza-Marinucci M, et al. Effects of two different probiotics on microflora, morphology, and morphometry of gut in organic laying hens. Poultry Science. 2016;**95**(11):2528-2535. DOI: 10.3382/PS/PEW164

[57] Sen S, Ingale SL, Kim JS, Kim KH, Kim YW, Khong C, et al. Effect of supplementation of *B. subtilis* LS 1-2 grown on citrus-juice waste and corn-soybean meal substrate on growth performance, nutrient retention, caecal microbiology and small intestinal morphology of broilers. Asian-Australasian Journal of Animal Sciences. 2011;**24**(8):1120-1127. DOI: 10.5713/AJAS.2011.10443

[58] Kazemi SA, Ahmadi H, Karimi Torshizi MA. Evaluating two multistrain probiotics on growth performance, intestinal morphology, lipid oxidation and ileal microflora in chickens. Journal of Animal Physiology and Animal Nutrition. 2019;**103**(5):1399-1407. DOI: 10.1111/jpn.13124

[59] Li G, Tong Y, Xiao Y, Huang S, Zhao T, Xia X. Probiotic *B. subtilis* contributes to the modulation of gut microbiota and blood metabolic profile of hosts. Comparative Biochemistry and Physiology Toxicology & Pharmacology: CBP. 2023;**272**:109712. DOI: 10.1016/J.CBPC.2023.109712

[60] Hu Y, Dun Y, Li S, Zhao S, Peng N, Liang Y. Effects of *B. subtilis* KN-42 on growth performance, diarrhea and faecal bacterial flora of weaned piglets. Asian-Australasian Journal of Animal Sciences. 2014;**27**(8):1131. DOI: 10.5713/AJAS.2013.13737

[61] Baker AA, Davis E, Spencer JD, Moser R, Rehberger T. The effect of a *Bacillus*-based direct-fed microbial supplemented to sows on the gastrointestinal microbiota of their neonatal piglets. Journal of Animal Science. 2013;**91**(7):3390-3399. DOI: 10.2527/JAS.2012-5821

[62] Wang H, Kim KP, Kim IH. Influence of *B. subtilis* GCB-13-001 on growth performance, nutrient digestibility, blood characteristics, faecal microbiota and faecal score in weanling pigs. Journal of Animal Physiology and Animal Nutrition. 2019;**103**(6):1919-1925. DOI: 10.1111/jpn.13199

[63] Zhang Q, Li J, Cao M, Li Y, Zhuo Y, Fang Z, et al. Dietary supplementation of *B. subtilis* PB6 improves sow reproductive performance and reduces piglet birth intervals. Animal Nutrition. 2020;**6**(3):278

[64] Lv L, Mu D, Du Y, Yan R, Jiang H. Mechanism of the immunomodulatory effect of the combination of live

Bifidobacterium, *Lactobacillus*, *Enterococcus*, and *Bacillus* on immunocompromised rats. Frontiers in Immunology. 2021;**12**:694344. DOI: 10.3389/FIMMU.2021.694344/

[65] Cogliati S, Clementi V, Francisco M, Crespo C, Argañaraz F, Grau R. *B. subtilis* delays neurodegeneration and behavioral impairment in the Alzheimer's disease model caenorhabditis elegans. Journal of Alzheimer's Disease. 2020;**73**(3):1035-1052. DOI: 10.3233/JAD-190837

[66] Goya ME, Xue F, Sampedro-Torres-Quevedo C, Arnaouteli S, Riquelme-Dominguez L, Romanowski A, et al. Probiotic *B. subtilis* protects against α-synuclein aggregation in *C. elegans*. Cell Reports. 2020;**30**(2):367. DOI: 10.1016/J.CELREP.2019.12.078

[67] Ayala FR, Bauman C, Cogliati S, Leñini C, Bartolini M, Grau R. Microbial flora, probiotics, *B. subtilis* and the search for a long and healthy human longevity. Microbial Cell. 2017;**4**(4):133. DOI: 10.15698/MIC2017.04.569

[68] Trotter RE, Vazquez AR, Grubb DS, Freedman KE, Grabos LE, Jones S, et al. *B. subtilis* DE111 intake may improve blood lipids and endothelial function in healthy adults. Beneficial Microbes. 2020;**11**(7):621-630. DOI: 10.3920/BM2020.0039

[69] Weng Y, Yao J, Sparks S, Wang KY. Nattokinase: An oral antithrombotic agent for the prevention of cardiovascular disease. International Journal of Molecular Sciences. 2017;**18**(3):523. DOI: 10.3390/IJMS18030523

[70] Cardinali N, Bauman C, Rodriguez Ayala F, Grau R. Two cases of type 2 diabetes mellitus successfully treated with probiotics. Clinical Case Reports. 2020;**8**(12):3119-3124. DOI: 10.1002/CCR3.3354

[71] Penet C, Kramer R, Little R, Spears JL, Parker J, Iyer JK, et al. A randomized, double-blind, placebo-controlled, parallel study evaluating the efficacy of *B. subtilis* MB40 to reduce abdominal discomfort, gas, and bloating. Alternative Therapies in Health and Medicine. 2021;**27**(S1):146-157

[72] Hatanaka M, Kanzato H, Tsuda R, Nadaoka I, Yasue M, Hoshino T, et al. Safety evaluation of the excessive intake of *B. subtilis* C-3102 in healthy Japanese adults: A randomized, placebo-controlled, double-blind, parallel-group, comparison trial. Toxicology Reports. 2020;**7**:46-58. DOI: 10.1016/J.TOXREP.2019.11.009

[73] Kordowski A, Tetzlaff-Lelleck VV, Speckmann B, Loh G, Künstner A, Schulz F, et al. A nutritional supplement based on a synbiotic combination of *B. subtilis* DSM 32315 and L-alanyl-L-glutamine improves glucose metabolism in healthy prediabetic subjects—A real-life post-marketing study. Frontiers in Nutrition. 2022;**9**:1001419. DOI: 10.3389/FNUT.2022.1001419/

[74] Toohey JC, Townsend JR, Johnson SB, Toy AM, Vantrease WC, Bender D, et al. Effects of probiotic (*B. subtilis*) supplementation during offseason resistance training in female division I athletes. Journal of Strength and Conditioning Research. 2020;**34**(11):3173-3181. DOI: 10.1519/JSC.0000000000002675

[75] Hanifi A, Culpepper T, Mai V, Anand A, Ford AL, Ukhanova M, et al. Evaluation of *B. subtilis* R0179 on gastrointestinal viability and general wellness: A randomised, double-blind, placebo-controlled trial in healthy adults. Beneficial Microbes. 2015;**6**(1):19-27. DOI: 10.3920/BM2014.0031

[76] Garvey SM, Mah E, Blonquist TM, Kaden VN, Spears JL. The probiotic *B.*

subtilis BS50 decreases gastrointestinal symptoms in healthy adults: A randomized, double-blind, placebo-controlled trial. Gut Microbes. 2022;**14**(1):2122668. DOI: 10.1080/19490976.2022.2122668

[77] Paytuví-Gallart A, Sanseverino W, Winger AM. Daily intake of probiotic strain *B. subtilis* DE111 supports a healthy microbiome in children attending day-care. Beneficial Microbes. 2020;**11**(7):611-620. DOI: 10.3920/BM2020.0022

[78] Tom Dieck H, Schön C, Wagner T, Pankoke HC, Fluegel M, Speckmann B. A synbiotic formulation comprising *B. subtilis* DSM 32315 and L-Alanyl-L-glutamine improves intestinal butyrate levels and lipid metabolism in healthy humans. Nutrients. 2021;**14**(1):143. DOI: 10.3390/NU14010143/S1

[79] Takimoto T, Hatanaka M, Hoshino T, Takara T, Tanaka K, Shimizu A, et al. Effect of *B. subtilis* C-3102 on bone mineral density in healthy postmenopausal Japanese women: A randomized, placebo-controlled, double-blind clinical trial. Bioscience of Microbiota, Food and Health. 2018;**37**(4):87-96. DOI: 10.12938/BMFH.18-006

[80] Zocco MA, Dal Verme LZ, Cremonini F, Piscaglia AC, Nista EC, Candelli M, et al. Efficacy of *Lactobacillus* GG in maintaining remission of ulcerative colitis. Alimentary Pharmacology and Therapeutics. 2006;**23**(11):1567-1574. DOI: 10.1111/J.1365-2036.2006.02927.X

[81] Szajewska H, Wanke M, Patro B. Meta-analysis: The effects of *L. rhamnosus* GG supplementation for the prevention of healthcare-associated diarrhoea in children. Alimentary Pharmacology and Therapeutics. 2011;**34**(9):1079-1087. DOI: 10.1111/J.1365-2036.2011.04837.X

[82] Doron S, Snydman DR, Gorbach SL. *Lactobacillus* GG: Bacteriology and clinical applications. Gastroenterology Clinics of North America. 2005;**34**(3): 483-498. DOI: 10.1016/J.GTC.2005.05.011

[83] Yan F, Polk DB. Probiotic bacterium prevents cytokine-induced apoptosis in intestinal epithelial cells. The Journal of Biological Chemistry. 2002;**277**(52):50959-50965

[84] Yan F, Cao H, Cover TL, Whitehead R, Washington MK, Polk DB. Soluble proteins produced by probiotic bacteria regulate intestinal epithelial cell survival and growth. Gastroenterology. 2007;**132**(2):562-575. DOI: 10.1053/J.GASTRO.2006.11.022

[85] Mattila-Sandholm T, Myllärinen P, Crittenden R, Mogensen G, Fondén R, Saarela M. Technological challenges for future probiotic foods. International Dairy Journal. 2002;**12**(2-3):173-182. DOI: 10.1016/S0958-6946(01)00099-1

[86] Marino M, Innocente N, Calligaris S, Maifreni M, Marangone A, Nicoli MC. Viability of probiotic *L. rhamnosus* in structured emulsions containing saturated monoglycerides. Journal of Functional Foods. 2017;**35**:51-59. DOI: 10.1016/J.JFF.2017.05.012

[87] Cutting SM, Hong HA, Baccigalupi L, Ricca E. Oral vaccine delivery by recombinant spore probiotics. International Reviews of Immunology. 2009;**28**(6):487-505. DOI: 10.3109/08830180903215605

[88] Zhou Z, Gong S, Yang Y, Guan R, Zhou S, Yao S, et al. Expression of *H. pylori* urease B on the surface of *B. subtilis* spores. Journal of Medical

Microbiology. 2015;**64**(Pt 1):104-110. DOI: 10.1099/JMM.0.076430-0

[89] Ciabattini A, Parigi R, Isticato R, Oggioni MR, Pozzi G. Oral priming of mice by recombinant spores of *B. subtilis*. Vaccine. 2004;**22**(31-32):4139-4143. DOI: 10.1016/J.VACCINE.2004.05.001

[90] Zhao G, Miao Y, Guo Y, Qiu H, Sun S, Kou Z, et al. Development of a heat-stable and orally delivered recombinant M2e-expressing *B. subtilis* spore-based influenza vaccine. Human Vaccines & Immunotherapeutics. 2014;**10**(12):3649. DOI: 10.4161/HV.36122

[91] Chan BCL, Li P, Tsang MSM, Sung JCC, Kwong KWY, Zheng T, et al. Creating a vaccine-like supplement against respiratory infection using recombinant *B. subtilis* spores expressing SARS-CoV-2 Spike Protein with natural products. Molecules. 2023;**28**(13):4996. DOI: 10.3390/MOLECULES28134996

[92] Malaguarnera G, Giordano M, Nunnari G, Bertino G, Malaguarnera M. Gut microbiota in alcoholic liver disease: Pathogenetic role and therapeutic perspectives. World Journal of Gastroenterology: WJG. 2014;**20**(44): 16639. DOI: 10.3748/WJG.V20.I44.16639

[93] Yang M, Hutchinson N, Ye N, Yin J, Guan M, Wang Z, et al. Engineered *B. subtilis* as oral probiotics to enhance clearance of blood lactate. bioRxiv. 2024:2023.11.30.569300. DOI: 10.1101/2023.11.30.569300

[94] Cai M, Wan J, Cai K, Song H, Wang Y, Sun W, et al. Understanding the contribution of lactate metabolism in cancer progress: A perspective from isomers. Cancers. 2022;**15**(1):87. DOI: 10.3390/CANCERS15010087

[95] Williamson DH, Lund P, Krebs HA. The redox state of free nicotinamide-adenine dinucleotide in the cytoplasm and mitochondria of rat liver. The Biochemical Journal. 1967;**103**(2):514-527. DOI: 10.1042/BJ1030514

[96] Adeva-Andany M, López-Ojén M, Funcasta-Calderón R, Ameneiros-Rodríguez E, Donapetry-García C, Vila-Altesor M, et al. Comprehensive review on lactate metabolism in human health. Mitochondrion. 2014;**17**:76-100. DOI: 10.1016/J.MITO.2014.05.007

[97] Nørlinger TS, Nielsen PM, Qi H, Mikkelsen E, Hansen K, Schmidt NH, et al. Hyperbaric oxygen therapy reduces renal lactate production. Physiological Reports. 2017;**5**(6):e13217. DOI: 10.14814/PHY2.13217

[98] Sada N, Lee S, Katsu T, Otsuki T, Inoue T. Epilepsy treatment: Targeting LDH enzymes with a stiripentol analog to treat epilepsy. Science. 2015;**347**(6228):1362-1367. DOI: 10.1126/SCIENCE.AAA1299

[99] Pucino V, Cucchi D, Mauro C. Lactate transporters as therapeutic targets in cancer and inflammatory diseases. Expert Opinion on Therapeutic Targets. 2018;**22**(9):735-743. DOI: 10.1080/14728222.2018.1511706

[100] Thornton PK. Livestock production: Recent trends, future prospects. Philosophical Transactions of the Royal Society of London. Series B, Biological Sciences. 2010;**365**(1554):2853-2867. DOI: 10.1098/RSTB.2010.0134

[101] Gadde U, Kim WH, Oh ST, Lillehoj HS. Alternatives to antibiotics for maximizing growth performance and feed efficiency in poultry: A review. Animal Health Research Reviews. 2017;**18**(1):26-45. DOI: 10.1017/S1466252316000207

[102] Castanon JIR. History of the use of antibiotic as growth promoters in European poultry feeds. Poultry Science. 2007;**86**(11):2466-2471. DOI: 10.3382/PS.2007-00249

[103] Imperial ICVJ, Ibana JA. Addressing the antibiotic resistance problem with probiotics: Reducing the risk of its double-edged sword effect. Frontiers in Microbiology. 2016;7:232849. DOI: 10.3389/FMICB.2016.01983/

[104] Ben Y, Fu C, Hu M, Liu L, Wong MH, Zheng C. Human health risk assessment of antibiotic resistance associated with antibiotic residues in the environment: A review. Environmental Research. 2019;**169**:483-493. DOI: 10.1016/J.ENVRES.2018.11.040

[105] Aarestrup FM. The livestock reservoir for antimicrobial resistance: A personal view on changing patterns of risks, effects of interventions and the way forward. Philosophical Transactions of the Royal Society, B: Biological Sciences. 2015;**370**(1670):20140085. DOI: 10.1098/RSTB.2014.0085

[106] Laxminarayan R, van Boeckel T, Teillant A, Laxminarayan R, van Boeckel T. The Economic Costs of Withdrawing Antimicrobial Growth Promoters from the Livestock Sector. OECD Food, Agriculture and Fisheries Papers. Paris: OECD; 2015. DOI: 10.1787/5js64kst5wvl-en

[107] Cheng G, Hao H, Xie S, Wang X, Dai M, Huang L, et al. Antibiotic alternatives: The substitution of antibiotics in animal husbandry. Frontiers in Microbiology. 2014;**5**:87626. DOI: 10.3389/FMICB.2014.00217/

[108] Yuan C, Ji X, Zhang Y, Liu X, Ding L, Li J, et al. Important role of *B. subtilis* as a probiotic and vaccine carrier in animal health maintenance. World Journal of Microbiology and Biotechnology. 2024;**40**(9):268. DOI: 10.1007/S11274-024-04065-0

[109] Colom J, Freitas D, Simon A, Brodkorb A, Buckley M, Deaton J, et al. Presence and germination of the probiotic *B. subtilis* DE111® in the human small intestinal tract: A randomized, crossover, double-blind, and placebo-controlled study. Frontiers in Microbiology. 2021;**12**:715863. DOI: 10.3389/fmicb.2021.715863

[110] Latorre JD, Hernandez-Velasco X, Kallapura G, Menconi A, Pumford NR, Morgan MJ, et al. Evaluation of germination, distribution, and persistence of *B. subtilis* spores through the gastrointestinal tract of chickens. Poultry Science. 2014;**93**(7):1793-1800. DOI: 10.3382/ps.2013-03809

[111] Saravanakumar S, Prabakaran NN, Ashokkumar R, Jamuna S. Unlocking the gut's treasure: Lipase-producing *B. subtilis* probiotic from the intestine of microstomus kitt (Lemon sole). Applied Biochemistry and Biotechnology. 2024;**196**(7):4273-4286. DOI: 10.1007/s12010-023-04749-7

[112] Lee KW, Lillehoj HS, Jang SI, Lee SH. Effects of salinomycin and *B. subtilis* on growth performance and immune responses in broiler chickens. Research in Veterinary Science. 2014;**97**(2):304-308. DOI: 10.1016/J.RVSC.2014.07.021

[113] Lee Y, Park I, Wickramasuriya SS, Lillehoj HS. *B. subtilis* expressing chicken NK-2 peptide enhances the efficacy of EF-1α vaccination in eimeria maxima-challenged broiler chickens. Animals. 2023;**13**(8):1383. DOI: 10.3390/ANI13081383

[114] Hong HA, Huang JM, Khaneja R, Hiep L-v, Urdaci MC, Cutting SM. The

safety of *B. subtilis* and *B. indicus* as food probiotics. Journal of Applied Microbiology. 2008;**105**(2):510-520. DOI: 10.1111/J.1365-2672.2008.03773.X

[115] Chen B, Yang Y, Wang Z, Dai X, Cao Y, Zhang M, et al. Surface display of duck hepatitis a virus type 1 VP1 protein on *B. subtilis* spores elicits specific systemic and mucosal immune responses on mice. Probiotics and Antimicrobial Proteins. 13 Jul 2024. DOI: 10.1007/S12602-024-10323-2

[116] Li J, Yang M, Chen B, Wang Z, Cao Y, Yang Y, et al. Evaluation of the immunity responses in mice to recombinant *B. subtilis* displaying Newcastle Disease Virus HN Protein truncations. Microorganisms. 2024;**12**(3):439. DOI: 10.3390/MICROORGANISMS12030439/S1

[117] Guo K, Huang A, Lee O. Engineering of a novel anti-dioxin *B. subtilis* probiotic for poultry feed. Undergraduate Research in Natural and Clinical Science and Technology Journal. 2020;**4**(1-11):1-8. DOI: 10.26685/URNCST.190

[118] Merino-Guzmán R, Latorre JD, Delgado R, Hernandez-Velasco X, Wolfenden AD, Teague KD, et al. Comparison of total immunoglobulin A levels in different samples in Leghorn and broiler chickens. Asian Pacific Journal of Tropical Biomedicine. 2017;**7**(2):116-120. DOI: 10.1016/J.APJTB.2016.11.021

[119] Bahaddad SA, Almalki MHK, Alghamdi OA, Sohrab SS, Yasir M, Azhar EI, et al. *Bacillus* species as direct-fed microbial antibiotic alternatives for monogastric production. Probiotics and Antimicrobial Proteins. 2023;**15**(1):1-16. DOI: 10.1007/S12602-022-09909-5

[120] Xu J, Zhong F, Zhang Y, Zhang J, Huo S, Lin H, et al. Construction of *B. subtilis* strain engineered for expression of porcine β-defensin-2/cecropin P1 fusion antimicrobial peptides and its growth-promoting effect and antimicrobial activity. Asian-Australasian Journal of Animal Sciences. 2017;**30**(4):576. DOI: 10.5713/AJAS.16.0207

[121] Jung K, Saif LJ. Goblet cell depletion in small intestinal villous and crypt epithelium of conventional nursing and weaned pigs infected with porcine epidemic diarrhea virus. Research in Veterinary Science. 2017;**110**:12-15. DOI: 10.1016/J.RVSC.2016.10.009

[122] Gallien S, Moro A, Lediguerher G, Catinot V, Paboeuf F, Bigault L, et al. Evidence of porcine epidemic diarrhea virus (PEDV) shedding in semen from infected specific pathogen-free boars. Veterinary Research. 2018;**49**(1):1-9. DOI: 10.1186/S13567-018-0505-2/

[123] Niederwerder MC, Hesse RA. Swine enteric coronavirus disease: A review of 4 years with porcine epidemic diarrhoea virus and porcine deltacoronavirus in the United States and Canada. Transboundary and Emerging Diseases. 2018;**65**(3):660. DOI: 10.1111/TBED.12823

[124] Crawford K, Lager KM, Kulshreshtha V, Miller LC, Faaberg KS. Status of vaccines for porcine epidemic diarrhea virus in the United States and Canada. Virus Research. 2016;**226**:108-116. DOI: 10.1016/J.VIRUSRES.2016.08.005

[125] Yu M, Wang L, Ma S, Wang X, Wang Y, Xiao Y, et al. Immunogenicity of eGFP-marked recombinant *L. casei* against transmissible gastroenteritis virus and porcine epidemic diarrhea virus. Viruses. 2017;**9**(10):274. DOI: 10.3390/V9100274

[126] Liu P, Zhao J, Guo P, Lu W, Geng Z, Levesque CL, et al. Dietary corn bran

fermented by *B. subtilis* MA139 decreased gut cellulolytic bacteria and microbiota diversity in finishing pigs. Frontiers in Cellular and Infection Microbiology. 2017;**7**:300118. DOI: 10.3389/FCIMB.2017.00526/

[127] Wang J, Huang L, Mou C, Zhang E, Wang Y, Cao Y, et al. Mucosal immune responses induced by oral administration recombinant *B. subtilis* expressing the COE antigen of PEDV in newborn piglets. Bioscience Reports. 2019;**39**(3):BSR20182028. DOI: 10.1186/S12934-019-1151-8/

[128] Bjerre K, Cantor MD, Nørgaard J-v, Poulsen HD, Blaabjerg K, Canibe N, et al. Development of *B. subtilis* mutants to produce tryptophan in pigs. Biotechnology Letters. 2017;**39**(2):289-295. DOI: 10.1007/S10529-016-2245-6

[129] Peng H, Wang JQ, Kang HY, Dong SH, Sun P, Bu DP, et al. Effect of feeding *B. subtilis* natto fermentation product on milk production and composition, blood metabolites and rumen fermentation in early lactation dairy cows. Journal of Animal Physiology and Animal Nutrition. 2012;**96**(3):506-512. DOI: 10.1111/J.1439-0396.2011.01173.X

[130] Xu H, Huang W, Hou Q, Kwok L-y, Sun Z, Ma H, et al. The effects of probiotics administration on the milk production, milk components and fecal bacteria microbiota of dairy cows. Science Bulletin. 2017;**62**(11):767-774. DOI: 10.1016/J.SCIB.2017.04.019

[131] Sun P, Wang JQ, Deng LF. Effects of *B. subtilis* natto on milk production, rumen fermentation and ruminal microbiome of dairy cows. Animal. 2013;**7**(2):216-222. DOI: 10.1017/S1751731112001188

[132] Al Mamun MA, Sandeman M, Rayment P, Brook-Carter P, Scholes E, Kasinadhuni N, et al. Variation in gut bacterial composition is associated with *H. contortus* parasite infection of sheep. Animal Microbiome. 2020;**2**(1):1-14. DOI: 10.1186/S42523-020-0021-3/

[133] Xiang H, Fang Y, Tan Z, Zhong R. Haemonchus contortus infection alters gastrointestinal microbial community composition, protein digestion and amino acid allocations in lambs. Frontiers in Microbiology. 2022;**12**:797746. DOI: 10.3389/FMICB.2021.797746/

[134] Yang Y, Zhang G, Wu J, Chen X, Tong D, Yang Y, et al. Recombinant HcGAPDH protein expressed on probiotic *B. subtilis* spores protects sheep from *H. contortus* infection by inducing both humoral and cell-mediated responses. mSystems. 2020;**5**(3):e00112-20. DOI: 10.1128/MSYSTEMS.00239-20

[135] Yánez-Mendizábal V, Zeriouh H, Viñas I, Torres R, Usall J, de Vicente A, et al. Biological control of peach brown rot (*Monilinia* spp.) by *B. subtilis* CPA-8 is based on production of fengycin-like lipopeptides. European Journal of Plant Pathology. 2012;**132**(4):609-619. DOI: 10.1007/S10658-011-9905-0/

[136] Maksimov I-v, Singh BP, Cherepanova EA, Burkhanova GF, Khairullin RM. Prospects and applications of lipopeptide-producing bacteria for plant protection (review). Applied Biochemistry and Microbiology. 2020;**56**(1):15-28. DOI: 10.1134/S0003683820010135

[137] Mahapatra S, Yadav R, Ramakrishna W. *B. subtilis* impact on plant growth, soil health and environment: Dr. Jekyll and Mr. Hyde. Journal of Applied Microbiology. 2022;**132**(5):3543-3562. DOI: 10.1111/JAM.15480

[138] Qiu F, Liu W, Chen L, Wang Y, Ma Y, Lyu Q, et al. *B. subtilis* biofertilizer application reduces chemical fertilization and improves fruit quality in fertigated Tarocco blood orange groves. Scientia Horticulturae. 2021;**281**:110004. DOI: 10.1016/J.SCIENTA.2021.110004

[139] Rostami A, Hinc K, Goshadrou F, Shali A, Bayat M, Hassanzadeh M, et al. Display of *B. pumilus* chitinase on the surface of *B. subtilis* spore as a potential biopesticide. Pesticide Biochemistry and Physiology. 2017;**140**:17-23. DOI: 10.1016/J.PESTBP.2017.05.008

[140] Talley NJ. Functional gastrointestinal disorders as a public health problem. Neurogastroenterology and Motility. 2008;**20**(Suppl. 1):121-129. DOI: 10.1111/j.1365-2982.2008.01097.x

[141] Ouwehand AC, Forssten S, Hibberd AA, Lyra A, Stahl B. Probiotic approach to prevent antibiotic resistance. Annals of Medicine. 2016;**48**(4):246-255. DOI: 10.3109/07853890.2016.1161232

[142] Ishaque SM, Khosruzzaman SM, Ahmed DS, Sah MP. A randomized placebo-controlled clinical trial of a multi-strain probiotic formulation (Bio-Kult®) in the management of diarrhea-predominant irritable bowel syndrome. BMC Gastroenterology. 2018;**18**(1):71. DOI: 10.1186/s12876-018-0788-9

[143] Moskovicz V, Ben-El R, Horev G, Mizrahi B. Skin microbiota dynamics following *B. subtilis* formulation challenge: An in vivo study in mice. BMC Microbiology. 2021;**21**(1):231. DOI: 10.1186/s12866-021-02295-y

[144] Ben David N, Mafi M, Nyska A, Gross A, Greiner A, Mizrahi B. *B. subtilis* in PVA microparticles for treating open wounds. ACS Omega. 2021;**6**(21):13647-13653. DOI: 10.1021/acsomega.1c00790

[145] Sarkar A, Lehto SM, Harty S, Dinan TG, Cryan JF, Burnet PWJ. Psychobiotics and the manipulation of bacteria–gut–brain signals. Trends in Neurosciences. 2016;**39**(11):763. DOI: 10.1016/j.tins.2016.09.002

[146] Carding S, Verbeke K, Vipond DT, Corfe BM, Owen LJ. Dysbiosis of the gut microbiota in disease. Microbial Ecology in Health and Disease. 2015;**26**:26191. DOI: 10.3402/mehd.v26.26191

[147] Luang-In V, Katisart T, Konsue A, Nudmamud-Thanoi S, Narbad A, Saengha W, et al. Psychobiotic effects of multi-strain probiotics originated from Thai fermented foods in a rat model. Food Science of Animal Resources. 2020;**40**(6):1014. DOI: 10.5851/kosfa.2020.e72

[148] Cheng HW, Jiang S, Hu J. Gut-Brain Axis: Probiotic, Bacillus subtilis, Prevents Aggression via the Modification of the Central Serotonergic System [Internet]. Oral Health by Using Probiotic Products. London: IntechOpen; 2019. DOI: 10.5772/intechopen.86775

[149] Jiang S, Hu JY, Cheng HW. The impact of probiotic *B. subtilis* on injurious behavior in laying hens. Animals. 2022;**12**(7):870. DOI: 10.3390/ani12070870

[150] Wang H, Huang J, Sun L, Xu F, Zhang W, Zhan J. An efficient process for co-production of γ-aminobutyric acid and probiotic *B. subtilis* cells. Food Science and Biotechnology. 2019;**28**(1):155-163. DOI: 10.1007/s10068-018-0461-7

[151] Diez-Gutiérrez L, San Vicente L, Luis LJ, Villarán M d C, Chávarri M. Gamma-aminobutyric acid and probiotics: Multiple health benefits and their future in the global functional food and nutraceuticals market. Journal

of Functional Foods. 2020;**64**:103669. DOI: 10.1016/j.jff.2019.103669

[152] Gusarov I, Gautier L, Smolentseva O, Shamovsky I, Eremina S, Mironov A, et al. Bacterial nitric oxide extends the lifespan of *C. elegans*. Cell. 2013;**152**(4):818-830. DOI: 10.1016/j.cell.2012.12.043

[153] Arnaouteli S, Bamford NC, Stanley-Wall NR, Kovács ÁT. *B. subtilis* biofilm formation and social interactions. Nature Reviews. Microbiology. 2021;**19**(9):600-614. DOI: 10.1038/s41579-021-00540-9

[154] Donato V, Ayala FR, Cogliati S, Bauman C, Costa JG, Leñini C, et al. *B. subtilis* biofilm extends *C. elegans* longevity through downregulation of the insulin-like signalling pathway. Nature Communications. 2017;**8**:14332. DOI: 10.1038/ncomms14332

[155] Dhyani P, Goyal C, Dhull SB, Chauhan AK, Singh Saharan B, Harshita, et al. Psychobiotics for mitigation of neuro-degenerative diseases: Recent advancements. Molecular Nutrition & Food Research. 2024;**68**(13):e2300461. DOI: 10.1002/mnfr.202300461

[156] Khodavirdipour A, Chamanrokh P, Alikhani MY, Alikhani MS. Potential of *B. subtilis* against SARS-CoV-2—A sustainable drug development perspective. Frontiers in Microbiology. 2022;**13**:718786. DOI: 10.3389/fmicb.2022.718786

[157] Pinu FR, Beale DJ, Paten AM, Kouremenos K, Swarup S, Schirra HJ, et al. Systems biology and multi-omics integration: Viewpoints from the metabolomics research community. Metabolites. 2019;**9**(4):76. DOI: 10.3390/metabo9040076

[158] Mugwanda K, Hamese S, van Zyl WF, Prinsloo E, Plessis M d, Dicks LMT, et al. Recent advances in genetic tools for engineering probiotic lactic acid bacteria. Bioscience Reports. 2023;**43**(1):20211299. DOI: 10.1042/BSR20211299

[159] Appala, Naidu B, Kannan K, Santhosh Kumar DP, Oliver JWK, Abbott ZD. Lyophilized *B. subtilis* ZB183 spores: 90-day repeat dose oral (gavage) toxicity study in wistar rats. Hindawi Journal of Toxicology. 2019:3042108, p. 9. DOI: 10.1155/2019/3042108

[160] The Science Behind Pre-Alcohol: A Probiotic that Digests a Byproduct of Alcohol-Built with Genetic Engineering by a Team of Microbiologists [Internet]. Available from: https://zbiotics.com/pages/how-it-works [Accessed: September 25, 2024]

[161] Vijayakumar KN, Bamne SS, Crasta J, Kumar CS, Bhat RM, Shuster BM, et al. *B. subtilis* ZB423: 90-day repeat dose oral (gavage) toxicity study in wistar rats. Journal of Applied Toxicology. 2024;**44**(12):1874-1885. DOI: 10.1002/jat.4677

[162] The Science Behind Sugar-to-Fiber: A Probiotic that Turns Sugar into Fiber-Built with Genetic Engineering by a Team of Microbiologists [Internet]. Available from: https://zbiotics.com/pages/how-sugar-to-fiber-works [Accessed: September 25, 2024]

Chapter 3

Probiotic Applications of *Bacillus subtilis*

Mohamadsadegh Mohamadzadeh and Sakineh Abbaspour

Abstract

Probiotics are defined as live microorganisms that confer health advantages to their hosts. Some probiotics exhibit limitations, including susceptibility to temperature fluctuations, gastric acidity, and harsh conditions. This has led to exploring probiotics with higher intrinsic resistance and stability in harsh conditions. *Bacillus subtilis* has received attention due to its inherent probiotic properties, high resistance to harsh conditions, and ability to form spores. Significant progress has been made in understanding the probiotic potential of *B. subtilis*, uncovering various mechanisms of action. On the other hand, postbiotics secreted by *B. subtilis* have become an attractive field of interest for scientists. Numerous studies have validated the efficacy of *B. subtilis* as a dietary supplement for poultry and aquaculture. Furthermore, the Food and Drug Administration (FDA) has recognized *B. subtilis* as safe. These advantageous properties position *B. subtilis* as a highly promising probiotic for various applications.

Keywords: *Bacillus subtilis*, probiotic, postbiotic, food, drug

1. Introduction

Bacillus subtilis is a Gram-positive bacterium that can grow in aerobic and anaerobic conditions. It is commonly found in various natural environments and is recognized as being generally safe for both animals and humans [1, 2]. *B. subtilis* rapidly grows and requires few nutrients, enabling it to survive, colonize, and reproduce across diverse habitats easily. Consumption of *B. subtilis* can have beneficial effects and improve the health of the host cell [3]. Hence, *B. subtilis* is known as a probiotic. It can form spores through sporulation. The formation of bacterial spores helps the *B. subtilis* to survive in harsh conditions. *B. subtilis* probiotics can improve intestinal microbial flora, strengthen the immune system, and prevent intestinal inflammation through different mechanisms [4]. In patients diagnosed with diarrheal-type irritable bowel syndrome (IBS), *B. subtilis* spores have effectively diminished the disease's severity [5].

Bacillus subtilis probiotics can secrete various postbiotics, such as enzymes, short-chain fatty acids (SCFAs), vitamins, teichoic acids, and exopolysaccharides (EPSs). It produces a variety of active enzymes, such as protease, amylase, and cellulase, which efficiently break down proteins, starches, and fibers, thereby enhancing nutrient utilization by bacteria [6]. Using postbiotics derived from *B. subtilis* ACCC 11025 in the broiler chicks diet mitigated ammonia emissions from excreta. It diminished the prevalence of *Salmonella* while simultaneously promoting the growth of *Lactobacillus* bacteria [7].

The addition of probiotics into the diets of both humans and animals to promote health has garnered much attention. Notably, among many probiotics candidates, the *B. subtilis* exhibited a remarkable ability to form spores, enabling it to endure extreme environmental conditions. It is more suitable than other probiotic strains due to its non-pathogenic and non-toxic nature and capacity to produce antimicrobial compounds. *B. subtilis* provides many benefits to the host when added to the feed of aquatic, poultry, and farmed animals. Telli et al. [8] indicated that adding *B. subtilis* into the diet of Nile tilapia mitigated the stress levels related to high stocking density [8]. *B. subtilis* contributes to improved immune protection in broilers by neutralizing harmful pathogens and promoting the synthesis of natural antibodies [9]. The preventive administration of *B. subtilis* probiotics exhibited effects comparable to those of antibiotics, mitigating the stress associated with *Salmonella gallinarum* infection while enhancing growth performance, immune response, and the development of gut mucosa in broiler chickens [10].

Bacillus subtilis probiotic is used to treat various gastrointestinal (GI) diseases. Administration of *B. subtilis* DE111 at a dose of $1 \times 10^{\wedge 9}$ CFU (colony-forming units), taken as one capsule per day for four weeks, resulted in a significant reduction in total cholesterol and non-high-density lipoprotein cholesterol levels, improved endothelial function, and decreased low-density lipoprotein cholesterol [11]. *B. subtilis* spores can be used as a novel method to treat various diseases. High resistance when passing through the digestive system and enhancing gene expression are the advantages of *B. subtilis* in vaccine production.

In this chapter, after the definition of the probiotic and its mechanism of action, postbiotics secreted from *B. subtilis* are discussed. Then, the use of *B. subtilis* probiotics in human food, aquatic, poultry, and farmed animals, and finally, the use of *B. subtilis* in medicine and pharmaceuticals are discussed.

2. *Bacillus subtilis* as probiotics

The term "probiotic," originating from Latin, means to "for life." Long before the recognition of probiotic microorganisms, various fermented products—including kefir, cheese, beer, kumis, and bread were commonly utilized for both nutritional and therapeutic benefits [12]. In 2001, a committee of experts from the World Health Organization (WHO) established a definition that is still reliable today: "live microorganisms which, when consumed in adequate amounts, provide a health benefit to the host." In addition to various species within the *Lactobacillus* genus, numerous *Bacillus* species, particularly strains of *B. subtilis*, have been utilized as probiotics for both animals and humans [13, 14]. Notably, it is recognized as a widely used probiotic due to its metabolic properties, especially the ability to form spores. *Bacillus* spores' heat resistance contributes to products' stability above room temperature. It allows for the direct addition of spores into animal feeds, which are processed at temperatures ranging from 80 to 85°C. Furthermore, many spores can endure the acidic conditions of the stomach and the bile acids present in the small intestine. After germination, the effects of probiotics can be observed mainly in the upper and significantly in the lower intestine. Depending on the strain, *B. subtilis* probiotics can have different mechanisms of action, such as the ability to directly or indirectly inhibit pathogenic organisms. *B. subtilis* probiotics also enhance the intestinal barrier and immune response, produce metabolites that are selectively utilized by gut microbiota ("cross-feeding"), or release enzymes that render indigestible food accessible to both the host and microbiota. Protease, lipase, and amylase are the industry's most widely used enzymes produced by *B. subtilis* [15, 16].

2.1 *B. subtilis* safety

Bacillus subtilis is classified as safe by the Food and Drug Administration (FDA), indicating that it poses no harm to human health. Furthermore, the European Food Safety Authority (EFSA) has also deemed this species safe under its Qualified Presumption of Safety (QPS). Consequently, *B. subtilis* strains can be considered non-pathogenic bacteria for human consumption. Research conducted by the European Scientific Committee on Animal Nutrition has revealed no evidence of toxicity associated with *B. subtilis*. Both acute and chronic toxicity assessments in animal models have further corroborated the safety of these strains. Thus, *B. subtilis* can be considered an ideal multifunctional probiotic bacterium for humans [17].

2.2 *B. subtilis* spore formation

The formation of bacterial spores serves as a crucial adaptation for survival in harsh environmental conditions that threaten the viability of vegetative bacteria. The sporulation process is related to the availability of nutrients in the surrounding environment. When nutrient levels become low, the bacterium begins an irreversible growth program that culminates in spore formation due to nutrient deficiency. The endospore nucleus of the bacteria contains a compact and inactive chromosome. At the same time, the spore is enclosed in a coat rich in peptidoglycan and one or more protein layers, collectively known as the spore coat [18]. In response to nutrient deficiency, the vegetative cell undergoes a series of morphological changes that lead to the formation of a pro-spore in the sporangium mother cell. This forespore is finally released through the lysis of the mother cell. *B. subtilis* spores show significant resistance against extreme temperatures, pH levels, stomach acid, bile, and various solvents, thus maintaining their viability in the digestive system. In addition, *B. subtilis* spores can be stored for a long time without refrigeration [16].

2.3 Action mechanisms of *B. subtilis*

2.3.1 Modulation of intestinal microbiota

The gastrointestinal tract's microbiota is crucial for the host's digestion, immune response, nutrient absorption, metabolism, and overall development. A healthy balance of intestinal microbiota is vital for the well-being of all living organisms. It aids the host by assimilating dietary nutrients and modulating the development and functionality of the digestive and immune systems [19]. *B. subtilis* can modify the composition of the intestinal flora by promoting the growth of beneficial bacteria and simultaneously suppressing the growth of pathogenic bacteria. Lin et al. [20] indicated that the oral administration of *B. subtilis* led to a significant reduction in liver and intestinal pathological damage in infected mice. The probiotics effectively restored the diversity and composition of the intestinal microbiomes in these infected mice [20]. *B. subtilis* improved the microbiota-gut-blood system (MGBS) [21]. They positively influenced the physiological functions of the host by regulating circulating metabolites, including uric acid, arginine, serine, adenine, and pyridoxal [21]. The structural integrity of the intestine and the intestinal barrier's functionality are vital for digestion, nutrient uptake, and defense against pathogenic organisms. Research has shown that supplementing animal diets with *B. subtilis* increases ileal villus height and a favorable villus height to crypt depth ratio, consequently augmenting the area available for nutrient absorption [4, 22]. Research has demonstrated that oral administration of the probiotic *B. subtilis* to laying hens does not enhance egg production. However, it can promote a healthier microbiota profile, marked by an increased proportion of beneficial bacteria, and it also fortifies the intestinal barrier function by elevating the expression of tight junction proteins [23].

2.3.2 Prevention of intestinal inflammation

The potential of *B. subtilis* in the management of intestinal inflammation is noteworthy. This bacterium is crucial in preserving intestinal homeostasis and supporting host health. It is a candidate for addressing antibiotic-induced colitis, inflammatory bowel disease (IBD), such as Crohn's disease and ulcerative colitis [24, 25]. Li et al. [26] showed that *B. subtilis* RZ001 probiotic enhanced intestinal integrity and mitigated colitis symptoms by inhibiting the Notch signaling pathway and activating atonal homolog 1 (ATOH-1) [26]. The exopolysaccharide-rich fraction derived from *B. subtilis* J92 has the potential to function as a beneficial food component, enhancing intestinal barrier integrity and mitigating colonic inflammation associated with IBD [27].

2.3.3 Synthesis of antimicrobial agents

Bacillus subtilis in the gastrointestinal tract is crucial due to its elevated metabolic activity. It is known to produce a diversity of natural antimicrobial compounds. Lipopeptides are an essential group of antimicrobial compounds that include surfactin, fengycin, and iturin, all of which possess surfactant characteristics and exhibit antibacterial, antiviral, antifungal, and anti-inflammatory properties [28, 29]. *B. subtilis* synthesizes antibiotics, such as bacillaene and bacilysin, which reduce the viability of pathogenic microorganisms [30]. *B. subtilis* strains isolated from the feces of healthy chickens have shown effectiveness in inhibiting the growth of *Escherichia coli*, *Salmonella enterica*, and *Staphylococcus* species [31]. Furthermore, cultures of *B. subtilis* demonstrate antifungal properties against harmful fungi, including *Aspergillus brasiliensis*, *Colletotrichum gloeosporioides*, and *Botrytis cinerea* [30].

2.3.4 Improvement of immunostimulatory activity

Bacillus subtilis contributes to the defense against pathogens by stimulating non-specific and specific immune responses. Numerous studies conducted on human and animal models have demonstrated compelling evidence that the oral intake of *Bacillus* spores can boost the immune system. The spores of *B. subtilis* elicit specific humoral and cell-mediated immune reactions. Furthermore, the interaction between *B. subtilis* spores and macrophages is crucial for developing the host's innate and adaptive immune responses. Qiu et al. [22] exhibited that *B. subtilis* has the potential to induce elevated concentrations of serum immunoglobulins, specifically immunoglobulin A (IgA), immunoglobulin G (IgG), and immunoglobulin M (IgM) [22]. Consumption of dietary supplements containing *B. subtilis* resulted in elevated IgG and secretory immunoglobulin A (sIgA) concentrations within the ileal mucosa of laying hens [4]. Diets that include *B. subtilis* can activate toll-like receptor 4 (TLR4), producing pro-inflammatory cytokines, such as interleukin 1 beta (IL-1β), interleukin 6 (IL-6), and interleukin 8 (IL-8) [32].

3. *B. subtilis*' postbiotics

In recent years, postbiotics have gained attention as an attractive field of research in the context of health enhancement alongside probiotics. The International Scientific Society of Probiotics and Prebiotics (ISAPP) characterizes "postbiotics as a preparation of inanimate microorganisms and/or their components that confer a health benefit on the host" [33]. Various inactivation methods can be used to prepare inanimate microorganisms or their components. These methods ensure that the microorganisms are not alive and at the same time retain their beneficial properties. Inactivation can be accomplished using heat, as heat is a common method of inactivating microorganisms that effectively preserves their components for use as postbiotics. The utilization of ultraviolet (UV) light, ionizing radiation, ultrasound (US), supercritical carbon dioxide (CO_2), and detergents are non-thermal techniques for preparing inanimate microorganisms [34, 35].

Postbiotics include various substances, such as enzymes, short-chain fatty acids (SCFAs), vitamins, teichoic acids, exopolysaccharides (EPSs), fragments of cell walls, bacterial lysates (BLs), cell-free supernatants (CFSs), non-viable probiotics, and other metabolites generated by the gut microbiota [36, 37]. Postbiotics have the potential to modulate mucosal functions and enhance the host's immune response when added to animal feed [38]. Additionally, they can facilitate a balanced gut microbiota and improve nutrient absorption [39]. However, the beneficial impacts of various bacterial strains and postbiotic constituents can vary, indicating a need for further investigation to elucidate their mechanisms of action and refine their application across different species. The following section will explain the postbiotic types, and *B. subtilis* postbiotics will be discussed.

3.1 Enzymes

Enzymes are proteins that facilitate biochemical reactions by acting as catalysts. Microbial enzymes exhibit various biochemical, physiological, and regulatory roles within various biological processes. The contribution of industrial enzymes derived from *B. subtilis* to the biotechnology field is significant, facilitating progress in multiple products. Notably, *Bacillus* species' enzymes represent around 50% of the total enzyme market [40]. **Table 1** exhibits the types of enzymatic postbiotics secreted by *B. subtilis.*

These enzymes selectively minimize the need for harsh chemicals, energy consumption, and harmful environmental effects. Due to high stability and strength, they can be reused in multiple cycles. The potential of *B. subtilis* in industrial enzyme production and biocatalysis is still being investigated through genetic engineering and optimization of fermentation processes. Researchers are trying to increase the productivity of *B. subtilis* postbiotics, especially enzymes. These advances facilitate the development of more sustainable and economical biotechnological processes.

Enzymes	Application	Ref
Alpha acetolactate decarboxylase	Beverage	[41]
Alpha-amylase	Food, Textile, and Paper industries	[42, 43]
L-Asparaginase	Pharmaceutical	[44]
Beta-glucanase and beta-glucosidase	Beverage	[45, 46]
Cyclodextrin glucanotransferase	Food, Pharmaceutical, and Cosmetics	[47, 48]
Glutaminase	Food, Flavor	[49]
Lipases	Detergent	[50]
Protease	Food, Detergent, and Textile	[51, 52]
Penicillin acylase	Pharmaceutical	[53]
Pullulanase	Food and Beverage	[54]
Polygamma-glutamic acid	Food, Pharmaceutical, and Cosmetics	[55, 56]
Urease	Analysis, Beverage	[57]
Xylanases	Food and Beverage	[58]

Table 1.
The types of enzymatic postbiotics secreted by B. subtilis.

3.2 Short-chain fatty acids

SCFAs are the principal metabolites produced by gut bacteria. SCFAs are produced by the gut microbiota from the digestion of prebiotics, such as inulin and fructooligosaccharides. SCFAs consist of 1 to 6 carbon-based anionic compounds. An inactivated strain of *B. subtilis* BG01-4, rich in branched-chain fatty acids (BCFAs), was administered to individuals who reported having functional gastrointestinal disorders. BCFA has improved the gastrointestinal disorders [59]. Intestinal bacteria can produce acetate, propionate, and butyrate. Xu et al. [60] showed that adding *B. subtilis* to food supplements increases the amount of butyrate. No effect of increased propionate levels was observed [60]. *B. subtilis* can positively affect the growth rate, intestinal health, and immune response in chickens by increasing the concentration of butyric, propionic, isobutyric, and valeric acids in the colon and inhibiting inflammatory factors [9, 61]. *B. subtilis* R-179 enhanced their production of SCFAs [62]. *B. subtilis* fermentation extract treatment had the highest concentration of volatile fatty acids and total SCFAs compared with other treatments [63]. The fermentation of xylooligosaccharides produced by *B. subtilis* 3610 recorded the highest production of butyrate for human fecal inocula from two healthy donors (D1: 9.0 ± 0.6 mM; D2: 10.5 ± 0.8 mM) [64]. *B. subtilis* DSM 32315 combined with L-alanyl-L-glutamine increased butyrate as a postbiotic and butyrate producer [65].

3.3 Vitamins

Human microbiota, such as lactic acid bacteria and bifidobacteria, can synthesize vitamins [66]. Animals, plants, or fungi cannot synthesize vitamins. Fecal metagenomes proved the presence of enzymes for producing riboflavin, biotin, pantothenate, ascorbic acid, thiamine, folic acid, and vitamin K [67]. Various results show that the gut microbiome plays an essential role in the synthesis of vitamins [68].

Recently, the industrial production of riboflavin using the *B. subtilis* strain has significantly progressed. The *B. subtilis* strain has demonstrated the capability to produce riboflavin in high quantities, ensuring both quality and economic viability within white biotechnology [69]. Song et al. [70] increased the production of vitamin K2 by using N-methyl-N-nitro-N-nitrosoguanidine (NTG) and low-energy ion-beam implantation and optimizing the fermentation environment of *B. subtilis* [70]. Using *B. subtilis* with the fed-batch method in biofilm reactors, Mahdinia et al. [71] reached a concentration of 28.7 ± 0.3 mg/L of vitamin K [71]. Pyridoxal 5′-phosphate (PLP), the most critical form of vitamin B6, was produced using metabolic engineering from the 1-deoxy-D-xylulose-5-phosphate (DXP)-independent short pathway in *B. subtilis* [72].

3.4 Teichoic acids

Teichoic acids are a group of structurally varied anionic glycopolymers constituting key cell wall elements in Gram-positive bacteria, such as *B. subtilis*. Together with lipoteichoic acids, they can make up to 60% of bacteria's total cell wall mass. These components play crucial roles in the cell envelope, regulating cell wall rigidity and permeability and affecting the bacteria's morphology [73, 74]. Lipoteichoic acid derived from *B. subtilis* triggers a toll-like receptor 2 (TLR2)-dependent inflammatory response while simultaneously inducing the activation of mer receptor tyrosine kinase (MerTK) signaling to mitigate inflammation [75].

3.5 Exopolysaccharides (EPSs)

EPSs are primarily synthesized by lactic acid bacteria and comprise oligosaccharide units. These units include sugars, such as glucose, galactose, xylose, fructose, rhamnose, arabinose, and mannose. EPSs exhibit various biological activities, including cholesterol-lowering, antimutagenic, immunomodulatory, anti-inflammatory, antihypertensive, antitumor, antioxidant, antibacterial, antiviral, and digestive effects, which make them promising candidates for biomedical and pharmaceutical uses. In addition, EPSs are used in the food industry due to their properties as a stabilizer, emulsifier, and water-binding agent. The specific functions of EPSs can differ based on the microorganism responsible for their production, their chemical composition, and the context of host–microbe interactions. Secreted EPSs of *B. subtilis* diminished the infection caused by *Citrobacter rodentium* and stimulated the production of anti-inflammatory macrophages in the peritoneal cavity [76, 77]. Paik et al. [78] showed that EPSs derived from the probiotic *B. subtilis* reduced bacterial load and inflammation in mice with *S. aureus* bloodstream infection [78].

3.6 Non-viable probiotics

In recent years, research studies have revealed that non-viable probiotics, including cell-free extracts (CFEs), heat-inactivated bacteria (HIB), and cell-free supernatants (CFSs), demonstrate functions comparable to those of live bacteria. ISAPP has categorized these substances as postbiotics. Studies on *B. subtilis* LCBS1 showed that HIB and CFEs significantly improved feed efficiency. Apparent digestibility coefficients of protein increased, and jejunum pH significantly decreased in the HIB and CFE groups compared to the negative control group [79]. Kelwick et al. [80] exhibited that *B. subtilis* WB800N cell-free systems based on cellular extracts are ~72× more active than *B. subtilis* 168 systems [80]. *Bacillus* species, especially *B. subtilis* KU43, have CFEs with significant anti-biofilm activity against the food pathogen *Listeria monocytogenes* [81].

4. Application of *B. subtilis* in food products

Probiotic microorganisms are widely recognized for their positive impact on host health when administered in sufficient quantities. While they are primarily found in dairy products, their use is increasing in various commercial foods, including animal feed, aquaculture, fermented meats, fruit juices, cereals, baby foods, and ice cream. Among bacteria, *Lactobacillus* and *Bifidobacterium* are the most common dietary probiotics. However, they have little resistance to heat treatment. The diversity of probiotic foods is anticipated to increase with the utilization of probiotics that can withstand heat treatment and the conditions of the gastrointestinal system. Recently, *B. subtilis* has attracted the attention of researchers and food manufacturers due to its unique properties that combine the characteristics of both *Bacillus* and *Lactobacillus* genera. *B. subtilis* is a spore-forming bacterium known for its heat resistance and probiotic properties. The spores of *B. subtilis* demonstrate exceptional viability to changes in temperature, fluctuations in pH, and exposure to gastric acid and bile within the gastrointestinal tract [82]. Furthermore, extensive research has been conducted on the cost-effective microbial production of valuable industrial products, such as various enzymes derived from *B. subtilis*, which have applications in food production [83]. This section examines the importance of *B. subtilis* in the food industry for human and animal consumption. It summarizes various studies on *B. subtilis* products and their role as a probiotic in food applications. Research has revealed that *B. subtilis* constitutes a varied community within the gastrointestinal tract, possessing characteristics promoting colon survival. In addition to probiotic viability in the digestive system and the production process, the stability of probiotics in different food products is also essential.

The development of functional food that maintains the viability and functionality of probiotic microorganisms throughout processing and storage presents significant challenges. The survival of probiotics is not only affected by temperature, but also by various factors, such as food matrix composition, processing, and storage conditions. It is crucial to recognize that probiotics' stability, safety, and efficacy are determined by the particular strain rather than the species or genus. Several essential characteristics are important in the formulation of probiotics: the type and amount of probiotic used, the viability of the probiotic during processing, the stability during storage, the aqueous activity of the probiotic, the evaluation of the added cell populations, and the sensory acceptability of the final product [84]. Furthermore, elements, such as the food matrix and oxygen levels, can significantly affect the viability of probiotics. Many novel food products proposed as carriers for probiotics lack thorough data regarding the stability and longevity of probiotic cultures within the food matrix and the effects of processing and storage conditions on these microorganisms. Strains of *B. subtilis* HU58 and PXN21 were evaluated in whole-meal biscuits. Both strains demonstrated resilience during baking at 235°C for 8 minutes, experiencing merely a 1 log reduction in survivability. These results suggest that both *B. subtilis* spores can endure the baking process effectively, indicating significant potential for their addition to various functional food products [85]. Jafari et al. [86] investigated the viability of probiotic spores under different storage conditions. In this research, probiotics were inoculated into sausages before and after processing and stored in the refrigerator for 45 days. This study found no significant reduction in the viability of *B. subtilis* ATCC 15245 when the sausages were inoculated after processing. *B. subtilis* ATCC 15245 viability decreased from only 20.89 CFU/g [86]. Almada-Érix et al. [87] conducted an investigation involving eight distinct *Bacillus* strains recognized for their potential probiotic characteristics, assessing their performance in various food items, such as meatballs, crystallized pineapple, milk, ground black pepper, orange juice, bread, yogurt, and spaghetti. *B. subtilis* Bn1 demonstrated high resistance, exhibiting fewer than 10 CFU/g reductions across most evaluated processes. The other strains, specifically *B. subtilis* PXN21 and *B. subtilis* PB6, experienced under 10^2 CFU/g reductions. Notably, all strains maintained fewer than 10^2 CFU/g reductions in at least six tested processes. These findings suggest that *B. subtilis* probiotic strains possess considerable potential for integration into diverse food matrices [87].

4.1 Application of *B. subtilis* in aquaculture

Using probiotics in aquaculture as potential microbial agents to improve the health and well-being of different aquatic species has been considered [88]. Notably, probiotic strains of *Bacillus* can sporulate, enabling them to withstand harsh environmental conditions. In addition, these microorganisms, with their non-pathogenic and non-toxic nature when consumed by aquatic animals and their potential to synthesize antimicrobial compounds, make them more beneficial than other probiotics [89]. Numerous probiotic species within the *Bacillus* genus are presently utilized, with *B. subtilis* being one of the most extensively studied and commonly employed probiotics in aquaculture. This bacterium offers many advantageous effects, including enhancements in growth, nutrition, immune function, and disease resistance among aquatic organisms. *B. subtilis* operates through various distinct yet interconnected mechanisms, including competitive exclusion, synergistic, antagonistic, and immune stimulation [90]. **Table 2** shows some studies on the effect of *B. subtilis* probiotics on different aquatic species.

Effective water quality management is essential for optimizing production in intensive aquaculture systems. To achieve this, various strategies are employed to ensure that water quality parameters remain within ideal ranges. Bioremediation is a particularly effective and widely accepted method that has gained prominence in aquaculture through probiotics [95]. Several microorganisms have been investigated for their ability to reduce or eliminate toxic pollutants in aquatic environments, providing a cost-effective and sustainable solution. The role of bacteria in bioremediation has been well established, and *Bacillus* species have been particularly noted for the removal of organic waste, heavy metals, and other pollutants. Notably, *B. subtilis* is often used for wastewater treatment and effectively improves water quality indicators, such as chemical oxygen demand, dissolved oxygen, nitrite, phosphorus, and ammonia levels [96]. Samani et al. [97] showed that the probiotic *B. subtilis* significantly reduced total ammonium, nitrate, nitrite, turbidity, and bacterial counts in the effluent of common carp ponds within four days [97]. Zhang et al. [98] reported the improvement of water quality parameters after treatment with *B. subtilis SC02*. In addition, the bacterial community strain increased the proportion of *Proteobacteria* (45.0%), *Bacteroidetes* (21.9%), and *Actinobacteria* (21.9%) [98]. Furthermore, the direct addition of *B. subtilis* to rearing water has enhanced aquatic organisms' overall health and survival rates by rapidly degrading leftover feed and organic waste [99].

Strain	Aquatic species	Dose	Benefits	Reference
B. subtilis WB60	Fish species Nile tilapia, *Oreochromis niloticus*	$10^{7/8}$ CFU/g	It caused weight gain, superoxide dismutase activity, myeloperoxidase, lysozyme, specific growth rate, and feed efficiency. On the other hand, it also improved the length of intestinal and muscular villi.	[91]
B. subtilis NZ86	Nile tilapia, *O. niloticus*	1.07×10^4 CFU/g	Lysozyme function, respiratory burst, and cytokines improved.	[92]
B. subtilis Ch9	Grass carp (*Ctenopharyngodon idella*)	5×10^7 CFU/mL	*B. subtilis* inhibited the reduction of Ca^{2+}, Na^+, K^+, and Mg2+, ATPase activity, and the damage to intestinal mucosal barrier function and inflammation induced by *Aeromonas hydrophila*.	[93]
B. subtilis	Silver pomfret, *Pampus argentus*	10^8 CFU/g	Probiotics improved the activity of lipase, superoxide dismutase, protease, and amylase.	[94]

Table 2.
Studies on the effect of B. subtilis *probiotics on aquatic species.*

4.2 *B. subtilis* in farmed animal health

The use of *B. subtilis* probiotics in feeding various farmed animals has been of great interest in recent years. The poultry industry faces significant challenges due to strict regulations governing antibiotic growth promoters (AGPs) use in livestock production, alongside a notable shift in consumer preferences toward AGP-free meat. Probiotics, especially those from the genus *Bacillus*, have been considered a suitable alternative because their ability to form spores has many advantages over traditional probiotic options. Probiotics enhance poultry growth performance and play an essential role in regulating gut health and immune responses. Additionally, it reduces the release of harmful substances in feces, thereby contributing to environmental sustainability and minimizing the risk of cross-contamination [100]. The gastrointestinal tract's health is crucial for poultry's growth and performance. In broiler chickens, dietary supplements containing *B. subtilis* have been shown to increase the height of the ileal villi and improve the ratio of villus height to crypt depth. Additionally, these supplements help establish a balanced microbiota by diminishing harmful bacteria while promoting beneficial strains, enhancing both immune response and intestinal barrier function [32, 101].

Liu et al. [102] showed that adding *B. subtilis* C-3102 to the diet of laying breeders increased the fertilization rate, weight, hatchability, and egg quality indices, such as yolk color and eggshell thickness index [102]. *B. subtilis* shows significant antagonistic properties against *E. coli, Clostridium perfringens, Eimeria maxima*, and other pathogenic microorganisms. Research indicates that strains *B. subtilis* B21 and DSM 32315 can enhance the performance and intestinal well-being of broiler chickens suffering from necrotic enteritis induced by *C. perfringens* [103, 104]. The study by Cramer et al. [105] illustrated that feeding broilers with *B. subtilis* enhanced breast weight and reduced the oxidative deterioration of breast muscle [105]. Li et al. [106] showed that

Strain	Animal species	Dose	Benefits	Reference
B. subtilis	Striped catfish	Four different levels (0, 1×10^6, 1×10^8, 1×10^{10} CFU/g)	Enhanced the growth rate, antioxidant capacity, protein levels, and immune response to *S. aureus* in striped catfish.	[109]
B. subtilis HH2	Beagles	5.0×10^8 CFU/mL	The relative abundance of Deinococcus-Thermus in the fecal matter was diminished, enhancement of nonspecific immune responses, and mitigation of ETEC-induced injury to the intestinal mucosal	[110]
B. subtilis MRS11	Nile tilapia	1×10^8 CFU/g	Enhanced growth performance and Improved gut morphology, alongside an increased relative mRNA expression of immune genes, contributed to improved resistance against *Streptococcus iniae* pathogen.	[111]
B. subtilis C-3102	Holstein dairy cattle	3×10^9 CFU/cattle	Improved milk production efficiency, effectively restricted the colonization of *S. aureus*, and prevented microbial infections in the mammary glands.	[112]
B. subtilis E20	White shrimp	10^9 CFU kg/diet	Enhanced the digestibility of glutamine in dietary intake and increased immune system efficacy.	[113]

Table 3.
Studies on the effect of B. subtilis *probiotics on farmed animals.*

the antagonistic effects of *B. subtilis* L6 on *E. coli* were effected in ducks. Furthermore, *B. subtilis* influenced antioxidant levels and energy metabolism by activating ribosomal functions and signaling pathways associated with oxidative phosphorylation, thereby reducing the damage caused by *E. coli* infection in ducks [106].

In addition to the abundant use of *B. subtilis* in poultry farming, this bacterium can be useful for other farmed animals. *B. subtilis* is a bacterial species recognized for its ability to produce a wide array of antimicrobial compounds, surpassing other members of the *Bacillus* genus. Research has demonstrated its efficacy in inhibiting the influenza virus and managing acute intestinal infections and antibiotic-associated diarrhea [107, 108]. The positive impacts of *B. subtilis* on various animal species, excluding poultry, are detailed in **Table 3**.

5. Pharmaceutical and medical applications of *B. subtilis*

Research on pharmaceutical and medical applications of probiotic *B. subtilis* on humans has increased significantly in recent years. Research often emphasizes the effect of *B. subtilis* on people suffering from various intestinal infections and diseases, such as ulcerative colitis, antibiotic-associated diarrhea, irritable bowel syndrome, acute intestinal infections, and *Helicobacter pylori* eradication therapy. Additionally, studies have concentrated on infections of diverse origins and dysbiosis, particularly in infants and children [114, 115]. The findings of research involving strains of *B. subtilis* administered orally in encapsulated forms are summarized in **Table 4**, highlighting their effects on human gastrointestinal health, modifications to gastrointestinal microbiota, and other health-related parameters.

Strain	Study design	Dose	Benefits	Reference
B. subtilis BG01-4	Randomized, aged 18–75, n = 67, with a self-reported diagnosis of functional gastrointestinal disorders (FGIDs).	5×10^9 CFU/day	Compared to the placebo, the probiotic group showed marked improvements in clusters for constipation (18%), constipation (15%), indigestion (11%), and dyspepsia (10%).	[59]
B. subtilis BS50	Randomized, aged 30–65, n = 76, self-reported abdominal burping, bloating, and flatulence.	2×10^9 CFU 1 capsule/day	Improvement of one or more points in the Gastrointestinal Tract Questionnaire (GITQ) for symptoms of burping (44.7% versus 22.2%) and bloating (31.6% versus 13.9%) in comparison to the placebo group. However, no notable differences were observed between the groups regarding flatulence (47.4% versus 44.4%)	[116]
B. subtilis DE111	Randomized, aged 20–65, n = 44	1×10^9 CFU 1 capsule/day	The probiotic group exhibited an elevation in the populations of anti-inflammatory immune cells following stimulation of peripheral blood mononuclear cells (PBMCs) with lipopolysaccharide (LPS).	[117]
B. subtilis DE111	Randomized, college female athletes, n = 23	1×10^9 CFU 1 capsule/day	The DE111 probiotic group exhibited a notable decrease in body fat percentage (−2.05 ± 1.38%) compared to the placebo group (0.2 ± 1.6%).	[118]
B. subtilis MB40	Randomized, aged 18–75, n = 100, self-reported symptoms of abdominal discomfort and bloating	5×10^9 CFU 1 capsule/day	The male subgroup that received probiotics exhibited a decrease in the intensity of bloating and a reduction in the number of days experiencing abdominal discomfort and gas. Additionally, there was a 10% enhancement in the overall health score compared to the placebo group.	[119]
B. subtilis C-3102	Randomized, aged 20–79, n = 82, self-reported with loose stools.	2.2×10^9 CFU/day	Following the administration of probiotic treatment, there was a notable reduction in the frequency of stool production per day. Additionally, the quality of stool, assessed by BBC scores, exhibited a significant improvement.	[120]
B. subtilis DSM32315	Open-label, Healthy adults, n = 192	2×10^9 CFU 2 capsules/day	The levels of fasting glucose exhibited a significant reduction from pre-treatment to post-treatment. HbA1c levels showed a notable decrease from pre-treatment to post-treatment, recorded at 5.72% ± 0.27 versus 5.65% ± 0.30. Furthermore, there was an improvement in the postprandial glycemic response.	[121]

Table 4.
Applications of B. subtilis *probiotics in human studies.*

Enzymes secreted by *B. subtilis* are also widely used in pharmaceuticals. Polygamma-glutamic acid produced by *B. subtilis* can be an effective drug carrier in various medical applications [122, 123]. L-asparaginase serves as an enzyme utilized in the treatment of lymphoid cancers. Nonetheless, patients still need an L-asparaginase with better performance and fewer side effects. Bento et al. [44] exhibited that a newly engineered strain of *B. subtilis* for producing L-asparaginase holds promise for pharmaceutical applications [44]. Zhou et al. [47] used *B. subtilis* RIK1285 to produce penicillin acylase [47]. Penicillin acylase is a prominent biocatalyst in the industrial synthesis of semisynthetic beta-lactam antibiotics, including ampicillin, amoxicillin, and cephalosporins [124].

5.1 Spores of *B. subtilis* in vaccine and drug delivery

The spores of *B. subtilis* represent metabolically quiescent yet highly exceptionally durable cells that arise in the cytoplasm of vegetative cells when environmental conditions are conducive to growth or survival. These spores have been identified as a potential vaccine delivery mechanism, merging the benefits of both synthetic and live systems due to their distinctive physical, chemical, and biochemical characteristics [125]. As a live vector for orally administered antigens, *B. subtilis* spores present several advantages: they are capable of promoting gene expression, demonstrate enhanced resistance to the acidic or alkaline conditions of the gastrointestinal tract, and exhibit rapid germination and prolonged survival within phagocytic cells [125, 126]. Spores of *B. subtilis* were covalently bonded to curcumin and folate to form a composite known as Cur-FA-spore. This formulation was administered to the colon, where the drug was released after traversing the gastric barrier. The findings indicated that Spore-Cur-FA enhances the oral bioavailability of curcumin, which suppresses colon cancer cells [127]. A mucosal vaccine targeting *Mannheimia haemolytica*, a pathogen associated with bovine respiratory disease (BRD), has been developed. The formulation utilizes *B. subtilis* spores as an adjuvant [128]. Recombinant *B. subtilis* spores with the receptor-binding domain (RBD) of the SARS-CoV-2 (severe acute respiratory syndrome coronavirus 2) spike glycoprotein have been genetically fused to CotY or CotZ. This construct is suggested as a potential oral vaccine candidate against the SARS-CoV-2 virus [129].

5.2 *B. subtilis* and production of nanobodies

Nanobodies (Nbs), single-domain antibodies, represent a novel class of antibodies distinguished by their diminutive size, exceptional solubility, and remarkable thermal stability. Due to these advantageous characteristics, Nbs have garnered attention as potential diagnostic and therapeutic agents in oncology and infectious diseases and valuable tools in fundamental biological research [130, 131]. While the predominant method for producing Nbs involves using *E. coli*, this expression system poses challenges, such as the risk of endotoxin contamination, the necessity for bacterial lysis to extract intracellular Nbs, and the inherent vulnerability of *E. coli* to environmental stressors [132]. A new expression platform utilizing *B. subtilis* has been established to overcome these challenges, serving as a stable and efficient microbial factory for Nbs production. The spores of the engineered *B. subtilis* strains exhibit significant resistance to wet heat, acidic conditions, and desiccation. Remarkably, the spores can germinate, proliferate, and secrete Nbs following exposure to stressors without compromising yield or quality. Importantly, as a Gram-positive bacterium, *B. subtilis* is devoid of endotoxin, and its capacity to secrete Nbs directly into the culture supernatant simplifies the downstream purification process. These features may render *B. subtilis* spores particularly beneficial in creating diagnostic devices characterized by high portability and extended shelf life. Yang et al. [133] showed that four distinct nanobodies, which target small molecules such as caffeine and methotrexate or cell surface-associated protein antigens, such as programmed death ligand 1 (PD-L1) and cytotoxic T-lymphocyte-associated protein 4 (CTLA-4), can be efficiently produced and secreted by *B. subtilis* [133].

6. Conclusion

The utilization of *B. subtilis* probiotics in various organisms as food and drug supplements is rapidly expanding. When consumed in sufficient quantities, they can positively affect the host cell. Various studies have proven benefits, such as immune stimulation, antimicrobial activities, and modulation of microbial flora, in humans and animals. Various postbiotics secreted by *B. subtilis*, such as enzymes, SCFAs, and vitamins, have many uses in the food, drug, textile, and paper industries. On the other hand, the high stability of bacterial spores is a unique feature that keeps cells alive in various harsh conditions. Therefore, besides food and pharmaceutical use for humans, they are a suitable supplement for using aquatic, poultry, and farmed animals. Despite many research and industrial advances in recent years, more evaluations are needed to achieve other benefits of *B. subtilis* probiotics.

Conflict of interest

The authors declare no conflict of interest.

Thanks

We thank the best people in our lives, our parents; our success would not have been possible without their efforts.

Author details

Mohamadsadegh Mohamadzadeh* and Sakineh Abbaspour
Biotechnology Group, Faculty of Chemical Engineering, Tarbiat Modares University, Tehran, Iran

*Address all correspondence to: m.sadegh_m@yahoo.com

References

[1] Mohamadzadeh M, Ghiasi M, Aghamollaei H. Optimization of plasmid electrotransformation into *Bacillus subtilis* using an antibacterial peptide. Archives of Microbiology. 2024;**206**(3):116

[2] Errington J, Aart LTvd. Microbe profile: *Bacillus subtilis*: Model organism for cellular development, and industrial workhorse. Microbiology. 2020;**166**(5):425-427

[3] Stülke J et al. *Bacillus subtilis*, a swiss army knife in science and biotechnology. Journal of Bacteriology. 2023;**205**(5):e00102-e00123

[4] Chen X et al. Effects of dietary supplementation with *lactobacillus acidophilus* and *Bacillus subtilis* on mucosal immunity and intestinal barrier are associated with its modulation of gut metabolites and microbiota in late-phase laying hens. Probiotics and Antimicrobial Proteins. 2023;**15**(4):912-924

[5] Kasapoğlu BE. The effect of *Bacillus subtilis* on gut microbiota, disease severity, and inflammatory parameters in irritable bowel syndrome: A pilot study. Journal of Enterocolitis. 2022;**1**(3):56-60

[6] Danilova I, Sharipova M. The practical potential of bacilli and their enzymes for industrial production. Frontiers in Microbiology. 2020;**11**:1782

[7] Fang S et al. Effects of dietary supplementation of postbiotic derived from *Bacillus subtilis* ACCC 11025 on growth performance, meat yield, meat quality, excreta bacteria, and excreta ammonia emission of broiler chicks. Poultry Science. 2024;**103**(5):103444

[8] Telli GS et al. Dietary administration of *Bacillus subtilis* on hematology and non-specific immunity of Nile tilapia *Oreochromis niloticus* raised at different stocking densities. Fish & Shellfish Immunology. 2014;**39**(2):305-311

[9] Oladokun S, Adewole D. The effect of *Bacillus subtilis* and its delivery route on hatch and growth performance, blood biochemistry, immune status, gut morphology, and microbiota of broiler chickens. Poultry Science. 2023;**102**(4):102473

[10] Sikandar A et al. Effects of *Bacillus subtilis* on performance, immune system and gut in salmonella-challenged broilers. South African Journal of Animal Science. 2020;**50**(5):654-662

[11] Trotter R et al. Bacillus subtilis DE111 intake may improve blood lipids and endothelial function in healthy adults. Beneficial Microbes. 2020;**11**(7):621-630

[12] Ozen M, Dinleyici E. The history of probiotics: The untold story. Beneficial Microbes. 2015;**6**(2):159-165

[13] Mohamadzadeh M, Fazeli A, Shojaosadati SA. Polysaccharides and proteins-based bionanocomposites for microencapsulation of probiotics to improve stability and viability in the gastrointestinal tract: A review. International Journal of Biological Macromolecules. 2024;**259**(2):129287

[14] Jeon H-L et al. Probiotic characterization of *Bacillus subtilis* P223 isolated from kimchi. Food Science and Biotechnology. 2017;**26**:1641-1648

[15] Todorov SD et al. Bacillus spore-forming probiotics: Benefits with concerns? Critical Reviews in Microbiology. 2022;**48**(4):513-530

[16] Williams N, Weir TL. Spore-based probiotic *Bacillus subtilis*: Current applications in humans and future perspectives. Fermentation. 2024;**10**(2):78

[17] Brutscher LM et al. Preclinical safety assessment of *Bacillus subtilis* BS50 for probiotic and food applications. Microorganisms. 2022;**10**(5):1038

[18] Isticato R et al. *Bacillus subtilis* builds structurally and functionally different spores in response to the temperature of growth. Environmental Microbiology. 2020;**22**(1):170-182

[19] Mohamadzadeh M et al. Viability and stability evaluation of microencapsulated lactobacillus reuteri in polysaccharide-based bionanocomposite. Carbohydrate Polymers. 2024;**347**:122693

[20] Lin D et al. *Bacillus subtilis* attenuates hepatic and intestinal injuries and modulates gut microbiota and gene expression profiles in mice infected with *Schistosoma japonicum*. Frontiers in Cell and Developmental Biology. 2021;**9**:766205

[21] Li G et al. Probiotic *Bacillus subtilis* contributes to the modulation of gut microbiota and blood metabolic profile of hosts. Comparative Biochemistry and Physiology Part C: Toxicology & Pharmacology. 2023;**272**:109712

[22] Qiu K et al. Effects of dietary supplementation with *Bacillus subtilis*, as an alternative to antibiotics, on growth performance, serum immunity, and intestinal health in broiler chickens. Frontiers in Nutrition. 2021;**8**:786878

[23] Zhang G et al. Modulatory effects of *Bacillus subtilis* on the performance, morphology, cecal microbiota and gut barrier function of laying hens. Animals. 2021;**11**(6):1523

[24] Liu Y et al. Long-term and continuous administration of *Bacillus subtilis* during remission effectively maintains the remission of inflammatory bowel disease by protecting intestinal integrity, regulating epithelial proliferation, and reshaping microbial structure and function. Food & Function. 2021;**12**(5):2201-2210

[25] Zhang X et al. Prevention and alleviation of dextran sulfate sodium salt-induced inflammatory bowel disease in mice with *Bacillus subtilis*-fermented milk via inhibition of the inflammatory responses and regulation of the intestinal flora. Frontiers in Microbiology. 2021;**11**:622354

[26] Li Y et al. *Bacillus subtilis* RZ001 improves intestinal integrity and alleviates colitis by inhibiting the notch signalling pathway and activating ATOH-1. Pathogens and Disease. 2020;**78**(2):ftaa016

[27] Chung K-S et al. Protective effect of exopolysaccharide fraction from *Bacillus subtilis* against dextran sulfate sodium-induced colitis through maintenance of intestinal barrier and suppression of inflammatory responses. International Journal of Biological Macromolecules. 2021;**178**:363-372

[28] Caulier S et al. Overview of the antimicrobial compounds produced by members of the *Bacillus subtilis* group. Frontiers in Microbiology. 2019;**10**:302

[29] Ali N et al. Lipopeptide biosurfactants from *Bacillus spp.*: Types, production, biological activities, and applications in food. Journal of Food Quality. 2022;**2022**(1):3930112

[30] Erega A et al. Impact of *Bacillus subtilis* antibiotic *Bacilysin* and *Campylobacter jejuni* efflux pumps on pathogen survival in mixed

biofilms. Microbiology Spectrum. 2022;**10**(4):e02156-e02122

[31] Nguyen D-H, Le T, Nguyen H-T. Inhibition of *Salmonalla* enterica by a novel strain of *Bacillus subtilis* isolated from the faeces of healthy chickens. British Poultry Science. 2022;**63**(4):535-540

[32] Guo M et al. Dietary administration of the *Bacillus subtilis* enhances immune responses and disease resistance in chickens. Frontiers in Microbiology. 2020;**11**:1768

[33] Salminen S et al. The international scientific association of probiotics and prebiotics (ISAPP) consensus statement on the definition and scope of postbiotics. Nature Reviews Gastroenterology & Hepatology. 2021;**18**(9):649-667

[34] Zhong Y et al. Recent advances and potentiality of postbiotics in the food industry: Composition, inactivation methods, current applications in metabolic syndrome, and future trends. Critical Reviews in Food Science and Nutrition. 2024;**64**(17):5768-5792

[35] Boyte M-E et al. Probiotic and postbiotic analytical methods: A perspective of available enumeration techniques. Frontiers in Microbiology. 2023;**14**:1304621

[36] Mousavi Ghahfarrokhi SS et al. Management of cardiovascular diseases by short-chain fatty acid postbiotics. Current Nutrition Reports. 2024;**13**:1-20

[37] Vinderola G, Sanders ME, Salminen S. The concept of postbiotics. Food. 2022;**11**(8):1077

[38] Loh TC, Foo HL, Chang HM. Postbiotic metabolites of probiotics in animal feeding. Probiotic bacteria and postbiotic metabolites: Role in animal and human health. Microorganisms for Sustainability. 2021;**2**:179-190

[39] Liu Y, Wang J, Wu C. Modulation of gut microbiota and immune system by probiotics, pre-biotics, and post-biotics. Frontiers in Nutrition. 2022;**8**:634897

[40] Su Y et al. Bacillus subtilis: A universal cell factory for industry, agriculture, biomaterials and medicine. Microbial Cell Factories. 2020;**19**:1-12

[41] Oliveira RC et al. Production of the food enzyme Acetolactate decarboxylase (ALDC) from *Bacillus subtilis* ICA 56 using agro-industrial residues as feedstock. Fermentation. 2022;**8**(12):675

[42] Hu Q, Liu J. Production of α-amylase by *Bacillus subtilis* QM3 and its enzymatic properties. Open Access Library Journal. 2021;**8**(3):1-8

[43] Niyomukiza S et al. Isolation, purification and biochemical characterization of alkaline α-amylase from *Bacillus subtilis* strain W3SFR5 isolated from kitchen wastes. Applied Food Biotechnology. 2022;**10**(1):9-19

[44] Bento HB et al. Aliivibrio fischeri L-Asparaginase production by engineered *Bacillus subtilis*: A potential new biopharmaceutical. Bioprocess and Biosystems Engineering. 2022;**45**(10):1635-1644

[45] Šokarda Slavić M et al. Improvement of nutritional and bioactive properties of barley β-glucan-based food products using *Bacillus subtilis* 168 endo-β-1, 3-1, 4-glucanase. International Journal of Food Science & Technology. 2023;**58**(12):6825-6835

[46] Muradova M et al. Unlocking flavor potential using microbial β-glucosidases in food processing. Food. 2023;**12**(24):4484

[47] Zhou J et al. Efficient production of α-monoglucosyl hesperidin by cyclodextrin glucanotransferase from *Bacillus subtilis*. Applied Microbiology and Biotechnology. 2023;**107**(15):4803-4813

[48] Pardhi DS et al. Cyclodextrin glucanotransferase: Fundamentals and biotechnological implications. Applied Microbiology and Biotechnology. 2023;**107**(19):5899-5907

[49] Zhang Z et al. A novel method for high level production of protein glutaminase by sfGFP tag in *Bacillus subtilis*. International Journal of Biological Macromolecules. 2024;**262**:130092

[50] Irianto VS, Demirkan E, Cetinkaya AA. UV mutagenesis for lipase overproduction from *Bacillus cereus* ATA179, nutritional optimization, characterization and its usability in the detergent industry. Preparative Biochemistry & Biotechnology. 2024;**54**(7):918-931

[51] Alamnie G, Gessesse A, Andualem B. Production of surfactant-stable keratinolytic protease from *B. Subtilis* ES5 and its application as a detergent additive. Biocatalysis and agricultural. Biotechnology. 2023;**50**:102750

[52] Nguyen T, Nguyen CH. Determination of factors affecting the protease content generated in fermented soybean by *Bacillus subtilis* 1423. Energy Reports. 2020;**6**:831-836

[53] Rathinaswamy P et al. Purification and characterization of YxeI, a penicillin acylase from *Bacillus subtilis*. International Journal of Biological Macromolecules. 2012;**50**(1):25-30

[54] Zhang Y et al. Enhancement of pullulanase production from recombinant *Bacillus subtilis* by optimization of feeding strategy and fermentation conditions. AMB Express. 2020;**10**:1-9

[55] Hu L-x et al. Poly-γ-glutamic acid production by engineering a degU quorum-sensing circuit in *Bacillus subtilis*. ACS Synthetic Biology. 2022;**11**(12):4156-4170

[56] Elbanna K et al. Poly (γ) glutamic acid: A unique microbial biopolymer with diverse commercial applicability. Frontiers in Microbiology. 2024;**15**:1348411

[57] Liu Q et al. Food-grade expression of an iron-containing acid urease in *Bacillus subtilis*. Journal of Biotechnology. 2019;**293**:66-71

[58] Karunya SK et al. Optimization and partial purification of xylanase from *Bacillus subtilis*. Intl J. 2021;**12**(2):56-63

[59] Patch C et al. *Bacillus subtilis* (BG01-4TM) improves self-reported symptoms for constipation, indigestion, and dyspepsia: A phase 1/2A randomized controlled trial. Nutrients. 2023;**15**(21):4490

[60] Xu Y et al. Effects of *Bacillus subtilis* and *bacillus licheniformis* on growth performance, immunity, short chain fatty acid production, antioxidant capacity, and cecal microflora in broilers. Poultry Science. 2021;**100**(9):101358

[61] Shehata AM et al. In ovo inoculation of *Bacillus subtilis* and raffinose affects growth performance, cecal microbiota, volatile fatty acid, ileal morphology and gene expression, and sustainability of broiler chickens (*Gallus gallus*). Frontiers in Nutrition. 2022;**9**:903847

[62] Pi X et al. Effects of live combined *Bacillus subtilis* and *enterococcus faecium*

on gut microbiota composition in C57BL/6 mice and in humans. Frontiers in Cellular and Infection Microbiology. 2022;**12**:821662

[63] Oladokun S et al. *Bacillus subtilis* delivery route: Effect on growth performance, intestinal morphology, cecal short-chain fatty acid concentration, and cecal microbiota in broiler chickens. Poultry Science. 2021;**100**(3):100809

[64] Amorim C et al. In vitro assessment of prebiotic properties of xylooligosaccharides produced by *Bacillus subtilis* 3610. Carbohydrate Polymers. 2020;**229**:115460

[65] Tom Dieck H et al. A synbiotic formulation comprising *Bacillus subtilis* DSM 32315 and L-alanyl-L-glutamine improves intestinal butyrate levels and lipid metabolism in healthy humans. Nutrients. 2021;**14**(1):143

[66] Ayivi RD et al. Lactic acid bacteria: Food safety and human health applications. Dairy. 2020;**1**(3):202-232

[67] Arumugam M et al. Enterotypes of the human gut microbiome. Nature. 2011;**473**(7346):174-180

[68] Pham VT et al. Vitamins, the gut microbiome and gastrointestinal health in humans. Nutrition Research. 2021;**95**:35-53

[69] Chu R et al. Production of vitamin B2 (riboflavin) by *Bacillus subtilis*. Journal of Chemical Technology & Biotechnology. 2022;**97**(8):1941-1949

[70] Song J et al. Enhanced production of vitamin K2 from *Bacillus subtilis* (natto) by mutation and optimization of the fermentation medium. Brazilian Archives of Biology and Technology. 2014;**57**(04):606-612

[71] Mahdinia E, Demirci A, Berenjian A. Implementation of fed-batch strategies for vitamin K (menaquinone-7) production by *Bacillus subtilis* natto in biofilm reactors. Applied Microbiology and Biotechnology. 2018;**102**:9147-9157

[72] Richts B, Commichau FM. Underground metabolism facilitates the evolution of novel pathways for vitamin B6 biosynthesis. Applied Microbiology and Biotechnology. 2021;**105**:2297-2305

[73] Jeong G-J et al. Controlling biofilm and virulence properties of gram-positive bacteria by targeting wall teichoic acid and lipoteichoic acid. International Journal of Antimicrobial Agents. 2023;**62**(4):106941

[74] Han J et al. Insight into the structure, biosynthesis, isolation method and biological function of teichoic acid in different gram-positive microorganisms: A review. International Journal of Biological Macromolecules. 2023;**253**(5):126825

[75] Zhang B et al. Mer receptor tyrosine kinase negatively regulates lipoteichoic acid-induced inflammatory response via PI_3K/Akt and $SOCS_3$. Molecular Immunology. 2016;**76**:98-107

[76] Jones SE, Knight KL. *Bacillus subtilis*-mediated protection from Citrobacter rodentium-associated enteric disease requires espH and functional flagella. Infection and Immunity. 2012;**80**(2):710-719

[77] Paynich ML, Jones-Burrage SE, Knight KL. Exopolysaccharide from *Bacillus subtilis* induces anti-inflammatory M2 macrophages that prevent T cell–mediated disease. The Journal of Immunology. 2017;**198**(7):2689-2698

[78] Paik W, Alonzo F III, Knight KL. Suppression of *Staphylococcus aureus* superantigen-independent interferon

gamma response by a probiotic polysaccharide. Infection and Immunity. 2020;**88**(4):10128

[79] Tao B et al. Postbiotics of *Bacillus subtilis* LCBS1 have beneficial effects on bullfrogs (*Lithobates catesbeianus*). Aquaculture. 2023;**574**:739699

[80] Kelwick R et al. Development of a *Bacillus subtilis* cell-free transcription-translation system for prototyping regulatory elements. Metabolic Engineering. 2016;**38**:370-381

[81] Park YJ et al. Cell-free supernatants of *Bacillus subtilis* and bacillus polyfermenticus inhibit listeria monocytogenes biofilm formation. Food Control. 2023;**144**:109387

[82] Lin P et al. Progress in research and application development of surface display technology using *Bacillus subtilis* spores. Applied Microbiology and Biotechnology. 2020;**104**:2319-2331

[83] Wang Y et al. Supplemental *Bacillus subtilis* DSM 29784 and enzymes, alone or in combination, as alternatives for antibiotics to improve growth performance, digestive enzyme activity, anti-oxidative status, immune response and the intestinal barrier of broiler chickens. British Journal of Nutrition. 2021;**125**(5):494-507

[84] Wang G et al. Characteristics of probiotic preparations and their applications. Food. 2022;**11**(16):2472

[85] Permpoonpattana P et al. Evaluation of *Bacillus subtilis* strains as probiotics and their potential as a food ingredient. Beneficial Microbes. 2012;**3**(2):127-136

[86] Jafari M et al. Probiotic bacillus: Fate during sausage processing and storage and influence of different culturing conditions on recovery of their spores. Food Research International. 2017;**95**:46-51

[87] Almada-Érix CN et al. Quantifying the impact of eight unit operations on the survival of eight bacillus strains with claimed probiotic properties. Food Research International. 2021;**142**:110191

[88] Amenyogbe E. Application of probiotics for sustainable and environment-friendly aquaculture management-a review. Cogent Food & Agriculture. 2023;**9**(1):2226425

[89] Kuebutornye FK et al. Mechanisms and the role of probiotic bacillus in mitigating fish pathogens in aquaculture. Fish Physiology and Biochemistry. 2020;**46**:819-841

[90] James G et al. Bacillus as an aquaculture friendly microbe. Aquaculture International. 2021;**29**:323-353

[91] Won S et al. Effects of *Bacillus subtilis* WB60 and Lactococcus lactis on growth, immune responses, histology and gene expression in Nile tilapia, *Oreochromis niloticus*. Microorganisms. 2020;**8**(1):1-15

[92] Galagarza OA et al. Modulation of innate immunity in Nile tilapia (*Oreochromis niloticus*) by dietary supplementation of *Bacillus subtilis* endospores. Fish & Shellfish Immunology. 2018;**83**:171-179

[93] Kong W et al. Effect of *Bacillus subtilis* on *Aeromonas hydrophila*-induced intestinal mucosal barrier function damage and inflammation in grass carp (*Ctenopharyngodon idella*). Scientific Reports. 2017;**7**(1):1588

[94] Gao Q et al. Effects of probiotics dietary supplementation on growth performance, innate immunity and

digestive enzymes of silver pomfret, Pampus argenteus. Indian Journal of Animal Research. 2016;**50**(6):936-941

[95] Hlordzi V et al. The use of bacillus species in maintenance of water quality in aquaculture: A review. Aquaculture Reports. 2020;**18**:100503

[96] Kalaycı Kara A et al. The investigation of bioremediation potential of *Bacillus subtilis* and *B. Thuringiensis* isolates under controlled conditions in freshwater. Archives of Microbiology. 2021;**203**:2075-2085

[97] Naderi Samani M et al. Effect of different concentration of profitable bacillus on bioremediation of common carp (*Cyprinus carpio*) pond discharge. Sustainable Aquaculture and Health Management Journal. 2016;**2**(2):44-54

[98] Zhang X et al. *Bacillus subtilis* $SC0_2$ supplementation causes alterations of the microbial diversity in grass carp water. World Journal of Microbiology and Biotechnology. 2013;**29**:1645-1653

[99] Nair AV et al. Evaluation of in vitro and in vivo potential of *Bacillus subtilis* MBTDCMFRI Ba37 as a candidate probiont in fish health management. Microbial Pathogenesis. 2021;**152**:104610

[100] Mazanko MS et al. Beneficial effects of spore-forming *bacillus* probiotic bacteria isolated from poultry microbiota on broilers' health, growth performance, and immune system. Frontiers in Veterinary Science. 2022;**9**:877360

[101] Liu Y et al. Effects of *Bacillus subtilis* and antibiotic growth promoters on the growth performance, intestinal function and gut microbiota of pullets from 0 to 6 weeks. Animal. 2020;**14**(8):1619-1628

[102] Liu X et al. Effects of *Bacillus subtilis* C-3102 on production, hatching performance, egg quality, serum antioxidant capacity and immune response of laying breeders. Journal of Animal Physiology and Animal Nutrition. 2019;**103**(1):182-190

[103] Musa BB et al. *Bacillus subtilis* B21 and *bacillus licheniformis* B26 improve intestinal health and performance of broiler chickens with *Clostridium perfringens*-induced necrotic enteritis. Journal of Animal Physiology and Animal Nutrition. 2019;**103**(4):1039-1049

[104] Sokale A et al. Effect of *Bacillus subtilis* DSM 32315 on the intestinal structural integrity and growth performance of broiler chickens under necrotic enteritis challenge. Poultry Science. 2019;**98**(11):5392-5400

[105] Cramer T et al. Effects of probiotic (*Bacillus subtilis*) supplementation on meat quality characteristics of breast muscle from broilers exposed to chronic heat stress. Poultry Science. 2018;**97**(9):3358-3368

[106] Li C et al. *Bacillus subtilis* protects the ducks from oxidative stress induced by *Escherichia coli*: Efficacy and molecular mechanism. Antioxidants. 2022;**11**(10):1951

[107] Ruiz Sella SR et al. *Bacillus subtilis* natto as a potential probiotic in animal nutrition. Critical Reviews in Biotechnology. 2021;**41**(3):355-369

[108] Winther K et al. *Bacillus subtilis*-597 induces changes in lung pathology and inflammation during influenza a virus infection in pigs. Veterinary Microbiology. 2024;**291**:110032

[109] Liaqat R et al. Effects of *Bacillus subtilis* as a single strain probiotic on growth, disease resistance and immune response of striped catfish

(*Pangasius hypophthalmus*). PLoS One. 2024;**19**(1):e0294949

[110] Yang J et al. Protective effects of *Bacillus subtilis* HH2 against oral enterotoxigenic *Escherichia coli* in beagles. Veterinary Sciences. 2023;**10**(7):432

[111] Büyükdeveci ME et al. Effects of two host-associated probiotics *Bacillus mojavensis* B191 and *Bacillus subtilis* MRS11 on growth performance, intestinal morphology, expression of immune-related genes and disease resistance of Nile tilapia (*Oreochromis niloticus*) against *streptococcus iniae*. Developmental & Comparative Immunology. 2023;**138**:104553

[112] Urakawa M et al. Prevention of mastitis in multiparous dairy cows with a previous history of mastitis by oral feeding with probiotic *Bacillus subtilis*. Animal Science Journal. 2022;**93**(1):e13764

[113] Chien C-C et al. Probiotic, *Bacillus subtilis* E20 alters the immunity of white shrimp, *Litopenaeus vannamei* via glutamine metabolism and hexosamine biosynthetic pathway. Fish & Shellfish Immunology. 2020;**98**:176-185

[114] Zhang R et al. Probiotic *Bacillus subtilis* LF11 protects intestinal epithelium against salmonella infection. Frontiers in Cellular and Infection Microbiology. 2022;**12**:837886

[115] Keikha M, Karbalaei M. Probiotics as the live microscopic fighters against helicobacter pylori gastric infections. BMC Gastroenterology. 2021;**21**:1-18

[116] Garvey SM et al. The probiotic *Bacillus subtilis* BS50 decreases gastrointestinal symptoms in healthy adults: A randomized, double-blind, placebo-controlled trial. Gut Microbes. 2022;**14**(1):2122668

[117] Freedman KE et al. Examining the gastrointestinal and immunomodulatory effects of the novel probiotic *Bacillus subtilis* DE111. International Journal of Molecular Sciences. 2021;**22**(5):2453

[118] Toohey JC et al. Effects of probiotic (*Bacillus subtilis*) supplementation during offseason resistance training in female division I athletes. The Journal of Strength & Conditioning Research. 2020;**34**(11):3173-3181

[119] Penet C et al. A randomized, double-blind, placebo-controlled, parallel study evaluating the efficacy of *Bacillus subtilis* MB40 to reduce abdominal discomfort, gas, and bloating. Alternative Therapies in Health and Medicine. 2021;**27**:146-157

[120] Hatanaka M et al. Effect of *Bacillus subtilis* C-3102 on loose stools in healthy volunteers. Beneficial Microbes. 2018;**9**(3):357-365

[121] Kordowski A et al. A nutritional supplement based on a synbiotic combination of *Bacillus subtilis* DSM 32315 and L-alanyl-L-glutamine improves glucose metabolism in healthy prediabetic subjects–a real-life post-marketing study. Frontiers in Nutrition. 2022;**9**:1001419

[122] Xavier JR et al. Optimized production of poly (γ-glutamic acid) (γ-PGA) using bacillus licheniformis and its application as cryoprotectant for probiotics. Biotechnology and Applied Biochemistry. 2020;**67**(6):892-902

[123] Halmschlag B et al. Poly-γ-glutamic acid production by *Bacillus subtilis* 168 using glucose as the sole carbon source: A metabolomic analysis. Journal of Bioscience and Bioengineering. 2020;**130**(3):272-282

[124] Cobos-Puc L et al. Classical and new pharmaceutical uses of

bacterial penicillin G acylase. Current Pharmaceutical Biotechnology. 2020;**21**(4):287-297

[125] Oh Y et al. *Bacillus subtilis* spore vaccines displaying protective antigen induce functional antibodies and protective potency. BMC Veterinary Research. 2020;**16**:1-10

[126] Saggese A et al. The bacterial spore as a mucosal vaccine delivery system. International Journal of Molecular Sciences. 2023;**24**(13):10880

[127] Yin L et al. Bacillus spore-based oral carriers loading curcumin for the therapy of colon cancer. Journal of Controlled Release. 2018;**271**:31-44

[128] Uddin MS et al. Development of a spore-based mucosal vaccine against the bovine respiratory pathogen *Mannheimia haemolytica*. Scientific Reports. 2023;**13**(1):12981

[129] Vetráková A et al. *Bacillus subtilis* spores displaying RBD domain of SARS-CoV-2 spike protein. Computational and Structural Biotechnology Journal. 2023;**21**:1550-1556

[130] Del Rio B et al. Lactic acid bacteria as a live delivery system for the in situ production of nanobodies in the human gastrointestinal tract. Frontiers in Microbiology. 2019;**9**:3179

[131] De Pauw T et al. Current status and future expectations of nanobodies in oncology trials. Expert Opinion on Investigational Drugs. 2023;**32**(8):705-721

[132] Lynch JP et al. Engineered *Escherichia coli* for the in situ secretion of therapeutic nanobodies in the gut. Cell Host & Microbe. 2023;**31**(4): 634-649. e8

[133] Yang M et al. Engineering *Bacillus subtilis* as a versatile and stable platform for production of nanobodies. Applied and Environmental Microbiology. 2020;**86**(8):e02938-e02919

Section 3

B. subtilis Therapeutical, Agricultural, and Environmental Applications

Chapter 4

Clinical and Therapeutic Potential of *Bacillus subtilis* Antimicrobial Peptides

Sajid Iqbal, Mehwish Malik, Bushra Mustafa and Hussnain Ahmed Janjua

Abstract

The bioactive peptides produced by *Bacillus subtilis* have garnered significant attention for their diverse bioactivities and promising therapeutic applications. These peptides exhibit broad-spectrum activity against bacterial, viral, fungal, and parasitic infections, making them potent candidates for treating drug-resistant pathogens. Further, these peptides exhibited anticancer activity by selectively targeting cancer cells, inducing apoptosis, and inhibiting tumor cell migration and invasion. Beyond their direct antimicrobial and anticancer properties, *B. subtilis* peptides also possess immunomodulatory effects, enhancing host immune responses and reducing inflammation. This dual role in both pathogen elimination and immune regulation expands their therapeutic potential, particularly for use in chronic infections and wound healing. To prevent these peptides from hydrolysis, biomaterial and liposome delivery systems have been designed to improve the stability and bioavailability of *B. subtilis* peptides. The key challenge in peptide-based drug discovery is the accurate prediction of peptide functionality and stability, given the complexity of peptide interactions with biological targets. Machine learning algorithms can be employed to design bioactive peptides with optimized therapeutic properties and can accelerate the identification of novel bioactive peptides with enhanced efficacy and specificity. Overall, this chapter demonstrates diverse mechanisms of action, therapeutic applications, immunomodulatory effects, and delivery systems for *B. subtilis* peptides.

Keywords: anticancer peptides, immunomodulatory peptides, antimicrobial peptides, peptide stability, peptide delivery systems

1. Introduction

Bacillus subtilis, a Gram-positive, spore-forming bacterium, has gained substantial attention over recent decades due to its prolific ability to produce a wide range of bioactive compounds [1]. These peptides are part of the natural defense mechanisms, enabling the producing bacteria to thrive in diverse environments, including soil,

IntechOpen

water, and even the human gut [2]. Among the antimicrobial agents produced by *B. subtilis*, its peptides stand out for their remarkable structural diversity and potent bioactivity, offering promising therapeutic applications. As the global health community faces an escalating antibiotic resistance crisis, there is an urgent need for new strategies to combat resistant pathogens, and *B. subtilis* peptides are emerging and promising sources of new, diverse peptides [3]. The peptides produced by *B. subtilis* exhibit unique modes of action, primarily targeting microbial cell membranes, leading to disruption and eventual cell death [4]. Their broad-spectrum activity against bacteria, fungi, and viruses and their ability to bypass conventional resistance mechanisms make them particularly attractive as alternatives or supplements to traditional antibiotics.

Further, *B. subtilis* peptides have shown various biological activities, such as immunomodulatory, anti-inflammatory, and even anticancer effects [5]. These activities expand their potential beyond simple pathogen elimination and open new avenues for therapeutic applications. For instance, *B. subtilis* peptides can play a critical role in wound healing by preventing infection and promoting tissue regeneration [6]. Their immunomodulatory effects help to reduce inflammation and enhance the host's defense mechanisms, which can be especially beneficial in treating chronic wounds or infections in immunocompromised patients [7]. One of the most exciting research areas regarding *B. subtilis* peptides is their potential use in cancer therapy. Recent studies have indicated that specific *B. subtilis* peptides can selectively target cancer cells while sparing healthy tissue [8]. These peptides can disrupt cancer cell membranes or interfere with essential metabolic processes, leading to cancer cell death. This selective cytotoxicity offers hope for new cancer treatments with fewer side effects compared to conventional chemotherapeutics [9]. Additionally, the ability of these peptides to induce apoptosis or necrosis in cancer cells provides a new approach to targeting tumors, particularly those resistant to other forms of treatment [10].

B. subtilis has a long history of safe use in food, pharmaceuticals, and probiotics, making it a favorable organism for the clinical development of peptide-based therapies. Its designation as a Generally Recognized as Safe (GRAS) organism by regulatory agencies highlights its low toxicity and well-established safety profile in humans. This biosafety, coupled with the robust peptide production capabilities, makes *B. subtilis* an ideal candidate for the large-scale production of therapeutic peptides [11].

2. *B. subtilis* peptides and their activities

B. subtilis produces diverse peptides with multifaceted functions. Several mechanisms have been suggested to explain the molecular mechanisms triggered by antimicrobial peptides (AMPs); however, it remains unclear which of these proposed mechanisms is responsible for their biological effects [12]. Various models exist, and the specific mechanism likely depends on factors such as the particular peptide, its concentration, and the type of target organism. Additionally, bacteria have been observed to respond to AMPs and can even evolve resistance to their toxic effects [13]. These molecules are highly diverse, making it difficult to classify them. Several factors can be considered, including the molecules' sources, biosynthetic machinery, properties, biological functions, three-dimensional structure, covalent bonding pattern, and molecular targets [14]. Here, various *B. subtilis* peptides are discussed with their bioactivities.

2.1 Anticancer peptides

Anticancer peptides (ACPs) produced by *B. subtilis* have emerged as promising therapeutic agents due to their selective cytotoxicity against cancer cells [15]. These peptides exert anticancer effects through various molecular mechanisms, including direct membrane disruption, apoptosis induction, metastasis inhibition, and immune response modulation [16]. Here, we analyze the molecular mechanisms of anticancer peptides produced by the *B. subtilis* group (**Figure 1**).

2.1.1 Cell membrane disruption

The primary mechanism by which *B. subtilis*-derived ACPs target cancer cells is through direct interaction with the cancer cell membrane. Cancer cell membranes have higher levels of negatively charged phospholipids, such as phosphatidylserine, and increased membrane fluidity compared to normal cells [17, 18]. These features make them more susceptible to cationic and amphipathic peptides produced by *Bacillus* species, including surfactin, fengycin, and iturin.

Surfactin: Surfactin, a cyclic lipopeptide produced by *B. subtilis*, disrupts the integrity of cancer cell membranes through its amphipathic structure [19]. Surfactin inserts itself into the membrane, forming pores or causing membrane thinning, which leads to leakage of cellular contents and eventual cell lysis. The higher anionic phospholipid content of cancer cell membranes enhances its interaction with the membrane, resulting in selective toxicity. Additionally, surfactin has been shown to trigger calcium-dependent pathways that exacerbate membrane destabilization, leading to necrosis in cancer cells [20].

Fengycin: Fengycin, another cyclic lipopeptide produced by *B. subtilis*, exhibits promising anticancer and antifungal properties [21]. Like surfactin, it targets the cell

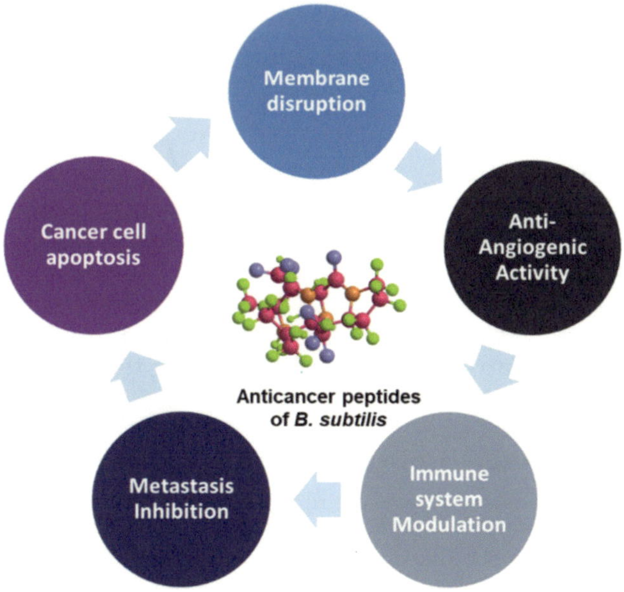

Figure 1.
Different mechanisms of B. subtilis*-derived anticancer peptides to target cancer cells.*

membrane of cancer cells. Fengycin preferentially binds to the lipid components of the cancer cell membrane, leading to structural disorganization and increased permeability [22]. This peptide is particularly effective against cells with high membrane cholesterol content, making it a potent agent against specific types of cancer cells, including those in leukemia [21].

2.1.2 Induction of apoptosis

Another significant mechanism of *B. subtilis*-derived ACPs is the induction of apoptosis, a programmed cell death process that is essential for eliminating cancer cells. These peptides can activate both intrinsic and extrinsic apoptotic pathways [16].

Iturin: Iturin, a lipopeptide produced by *B. subtilis*, induces apoptosis in cancer cells by disrupting mitochondrial function [23]. Iturin has been shown to depolarize the mitochondrial membrane, releasing cytochrome c into the cytoplasm [24]. This triggers the intrinsic (mitochondrial) apoptotic pathway by activating caspase-9, which then activates caspase-3, which cleaves cellular components and apoptosis. In addition to inducing mitochondrial damage, iturin also activates the extrinsic apoptotic pathway by binding to death receptors on the cancer cell surface, such as Fas and TNF receptors. This interaction leads to the activation of caspase-8, further amplifying the apoptotic signaling cascade. Through this dual apoptotic pathway, iturin effectively eliminates cancer cells while sparing normal cells [16, 25].

Mycosubtilin: Mycosubtilin, another peptide produced by *B. subtilis*, has demonstrated strong anticancer activity by promoting both apoptosis and autophagy in cancer cells. This lipopeptide activates the intrinsic apoptotic pathway by inducing mitochondrial dysfunction, activating caspases, and subsequent apoptosis [26]. Additionally, mycosubtilin can stimulate autophagy, a cellular degradation process that cancer cells can exploit for survival. However, excessive autophagy can lead to cell death, making mycosubtilin a dual-action peptide with the potential to suppress tumor growth [27].

2.1.3 Inhibition of metastasis

Metastasis, the spread of cancer cells from the primary tumor to distant organs, is a major cause of cancer-related mortality [28]. ACPs produced by *B. subtilis* have shown the ability to inhibit cancer cell migration and invasion, two critical steps in metastasis. For instance, Bacillomycin D, produced by *B. subtilis*, inhibits the metastasis of cancer cells by targeting matrix metalloproteinases (MMPs), enzymes that degrade the extracellular matrix and facilitate cancer cell invasion. Bacillomycin D explicitly downregulates the expression of MMP-2 and MMP-9, which are overexpressed in many aggressive cancers [29]. Moreover, Bacillomycin D prevents cancer cells from degrading the surrounding tissue by inhibiting these enzymes, thereby blocking their ability to invade and metastasize [30].

2.1.4 Modulation of the immune response

In addition to direct cytotoxic effects, Bacillus-derived ACPs can modulate the immune system to enhance the body's ability to fight cancer. These peptides act as immunomodulators, activating various immune system components, including macrophages, dendritic cells, and T cells, which can recognize and destroy cancer cells. Lantibiotics, a class of antimicrobial peptides produced by *Bacillus*, have shown the ability to enhance the immune response in cancer therapy [31]. These peptides stimulate the production of pro-inflammatory cytokines, such as TNF-α and IL-6, which activate immune cells and promote the recruitment of T cells to the tumor microenvironment. By enhancing the immune response, lantibiotics help eliminate cancer cells and reduce the likelihood of tumor recurrence [32].

2.1.5 Anti-angiogenic activity

Angiogenesis, the formation of new blood vessels, is essential for tumor growth and metastasis, as it provides the tumor with oxygen and nutrients. *B. subtilis* synthesized ACPs, demonstrating anti-angiogenic properties by inhibiting key pathways involved in blood vessel formation [33]. For example, surfactin produced by *B. subtilis* has been shown to inhibit the vascular endothelial growth factor (VEGF) pathway, which is a critical regulator of angiogenesis in cancer. By blocking VEGF signaling, surfactin reduces the formation of new blood vessels within the tumor, effectively starving the cancer cells and preventing further tumor growth. This anti-angiogenic activity and its cytotoxic effects make surfactin a highly potent anticancer agent [34].

2.2 Antibacterial peptides

Antibacterial peptides (AMPs) produced by *B. subtilis* are highly effective bioactive molecules that target and kill a wide range of bacterial pathogens through diverse molecular mechanisms. These mechanisms primarily include membrane disruption, inhibition of cell wall synthesis, interference with protein and nucleic acid synthesis, and disruption of intracellular processes. These peptides offer a promising alternative to conventional antibiotics due to their potency, stability, and reduced likelihood of developing resistance. Here, we describe the molecular mechanisms of *B. subtilis* antibacterial peptides with examples.

2.2.1 Membrane disruption

One of the most common mechanisms of action for *B. subtilis* producing AMPs is the disruption of bacterial membranes. These peptides often display amphipathic structures, which allow them to interact with the lipid bilayer of bacterial membranes, leading to pore formation, membrane destabilization, and cell lysis.

Surfactin: Surfactin is a well-known cyclic lipopeptide produced by *Bacillus subtilis*, characterized by its potent antibacterial activity. Its amphipathic nature enables it to insert into the bacterial membrane, where it interacts with membrane lipids, particularly phospholipids, causing increased membrane permeability. This leads to ion leakage, the proton motive force disruption, and eventual cell death. Surfactin is especially effective against Gram-positive bacteria, although it has also shown activity against some Gram-negative species [35]. The unique cyclic structure of surfactin enhances its ability to disrupt bacterial membranes, making it a potent antimicrobial agent [36].

Iturin A: Iturin A is another lipopeptide produced by *B. subtilis*, exhibiting strong antifungal and antibacterial activity. Iturin A targets the bacterial cell membrane by inserting itself into the lipid bilayer, where it forms transmembrane pores. These pores allow the uncontrolled passage of ions and molecules, leading to cell depolarization and cell death. Iturin A has a high affinity for ergosterol and cholesterol in fungal membranes but also exhibits activity against bacterial membranes by destabilizing their integrity. The broad-spectrum activity of iturin A makes it effective against resistant bacterial strains [37].

Fengycin: Fengycin is another cyclic lipopeptide produced by *Bacillus subtilis* that exhibits antibacterial activity, particularly against Gram-positive bacteria. It targets bacterial membranes by binding to specific phospholipids such as phosphatidylethanolamine, which is abundant in bacterial membranes. Fengycin's interaction with these lipids destabilizes the membrane, leading to increased permeability and leakage of cellular contents. Additionally, fengycin is particularly effective against biofilm-forming bacteria due to its ability to disrupt the membranes of biofilm-embedded cells [38].

2.2.2 Inhibition of cell wall synthesis

Several B. *subtilis*-derived peptides interfere with the synthesis of the bacterial cell wall, a crucial structural component, particularly in Gram-positive bacteria.

Bacilysin: Bacilysin is a small dipeptide produced by *Bacillus subtilis* that inhibits bacterial cell wall synthesis by targeting the enzymes involved in peptidoglycan formation [39]. Bacilysin specifically inhibits the enzyme MurA, which is responsible for the first step in peptidoglycan synthesis. By blocking this key enzymatic process, bacilysin prevents bacterial cell wall synthesis, leading to cell death. Bacilysin is highly effective against Gram-positive bacteria like *Staphylococcus aureus* and *Listeria monocytogenes* [40].

Subtilin: Subtilin, a lantibiotic produced by *Bacillus subtilis*, inhibits cell wall synthesis by binding to lipid II, a precursor molecule necessary for peptidoglycan biosynthesis. Lipid II is responsible for transporting peptidoglycan subunits across the cytoplasmic membrane to the growing cell wall. By binding to lipid II, subtilin prevents its incorporation into the cell wall, leading to cell lysis and death. Subtilin's mechanism is similar to that of vancomycin, but subtilin has the added ability to form pores in the bacterial membrane, further enhancing its antibacterial effects [41].

2.2.3 Disruption of nucleic acid and protein synthesis

B. subtilis peptides also can exert their antibacterial effects by disrupting bacterial DNA, RNA, and protein synthesis. These peptides can bind to nucleic acids or interact with ribosomes, preventing the transcription or translation of essential bacterial genes [42]. Bacitracin is a cyclic peptide produced by *B. subtilis* that inhibits bacterial protein synthesis by interfering with the recycling of undecaprenyl pyrophosphate, a lipid carrier involved in transporting peptidoglycan precursors across the cell membrane. By blocking the dephosphorylation of undecaprenyl pyrophosphate, bacitracin prevents bacterial cell wall formation and interrupts protein synthesis [43]. This dual mechanism makes bacitracin highly effective against Gram-positive bacteria, such as methicillin-resistant *Staphylococcus aureus* (MRSA).

2.2.4 Inhibition of biofilm formation

Biofilms protect bacteria from environmental stress and antimicrobial agents. Several B. *subtilis* peptides have been shown to prevent the formation of biofilms or disrupt existing biofilms, making bacteria more susceptible to antimicrobial treatment [44].

Plipastatin: Plipastatin, a peptide antibiotic produced by *B. subtilis*, has been shown to inhibit biofilm formation by preventing the adhesion of bacterial cells to surfaces. It interferes with the production of extracellular polymeric substances (EPS) necessary for biofilm integrity. Additionally, plipastatin can disrupt the structure of established biofilms by destabilizing the cell membranes of biofilm-embedded bacteria. This makes it a valuable agent in the treatment of chronic infections caused by biofilm-forming bacteria.

2.2.5 Interference with quorum sensing

Quorum sensing is a bacterial communication system that regulates gene expression in virulence, biofilm formation, and antibiotic resistance [45]. Some B. *subtilis* peptides have been shown to interfere with quorum-sensing pathways, reducing bacterial virulence and increasing susceptibility to antimicrobial agents [44]. For instance, Competence and Sporulation Factor (CSF), a small peptide produced by *B. subtilis*, interferes with quorum sensing by modulating the activity of signaling molecules involved in bacterial communication. CSF can inhibit the production of virulence factors and reduce biofilm formation by interfering with the regulatory pathways controlled by quorum sensing. This mechanism can weaken bacterial defenses and enhance the effectiveness of other antimicrobial treatments.

2.3 Antifungal peptides

Antifungal peptides (AFPs) produced by *B. subtilis* are bioactive molecules that exhibit potent antifungal activity through a variety of molecular mechanisms. These include disrupting the fungal cell membrane, inhibiting cell wall biosynthesis, and interfering with vital intracellular processes. Due to their high specificity for fungal cells, AFPs produced by *B. subtilis* have shown efficacy in combating fungal infections, including those caused by resistant strains, making them promising candidates for antifungal therapies. Research has explored these natural compounds for their capacity to inhibit pathogenic fungi in vitro by attaching to the plasma membrane and disrupting the lipid bilayer, thus interfering with different cellular processes [15, 46]. Structurally, these lipopeptides feature α-helix, β-hairpin, or sheet formations and include a β-hydroxy fatty acid, giving them the capability to inhibit several fungal species [15]. Below is a detailed exploration of the molecular mechanisms of *B. subtilis*-derived AFPs, along with specific examples.

2.3.1 Cell membrane disruption

The most common mechanism of antifungal action for AFPs derived from *B. subtilis* involves direct interaction with the fungal cell membrane. Many antifungal peptides have amphipathic structures that allow them to bind to fungal membrane components, resulting in membrane destabilization and cell lysis. Iturin A is one of the most well-known lipopeptides produced by *B. subtilis*. It specifically targets the fungal membrane by binding to ergosterol, a key sterol component of fungal cell membranes. Once bound to ergosterol, Iturin A inserts itself into the lipid bilayer, forming transmembrane pores. This leads to an increased permeability of the fungal membrane, causing ion leakage, osmotic imbalance, and eventual cell lysis. Iturins are effective against a wide variety of fungi, including Candida albicans, Aspergillus species, and Fusarium species.

Fengycin is another cyclic lipopeptide produced by *B. subtilis* and is primarily known for its strong antifungal activity. Like Iturin A, fengycin interacts with the fungal membrane by targeting specific lipids, particularly phosphatidylethanolamine and sterols such as ergosterol. Fengycin induces membrane destabilization and pore formation, leading to cell leakage and fungal death. Fengycin is particularly effective against filamentous fungi like *Aspergillus niger* and *Penicillium* species and is also effective against fungal phytopathogens. Recently, a new antifungal lipopeptide called AF3, isolated from a wild strain of *B. subtilis*, has been identified. AF3 exhibits strong antifungal activity, primarily targeting the cell membrane of *Candida albicans*, leading to membrane instability and disorder [47].

2.3.2 Inhibition of cell walls

Fungal cell walls are essential for maintaining the structural integrity of fungal cells, and disrupting cell wall biosynthesis can be lethal for fungi. Several B. *subtilis* peptides interfere with the synthesis of key components of the fungal cell wall, particularly chitin and β-glucan. Mycosubtilin, a member of the iturin family, exhibits potent antifungal activity by targeting the fungal cell wall. It primarily interferes with chitin synthesis, a major structural polysaccharide in the fungal cell wall. By inhibiting the enzymes involved in chitin biosynthesis, mycosubtilin prevents the formation of a functional cell wall, leading to fungal cell death. In addition to inhibiting cell wall biosynthesis, mycosubtilin also has membrane-disrupting properties similar to other lipopeptides, further enhancing its antifungal efficacy [48].

2.3.3 Interference with intracellular pathways

Some antifungal peptides produced by *B. subtilis* target the cell membrane or cell wall and disrupt key intracellular signaling pathways, leading to cell death. These peptides can interfere with fungal homeostasis by targeting enzymes, ion channels, and transporters. Bacillomycin D is a lipopeptide synthesized by *B. subtilis* and exhibits potent antifungal activity. In addition to disrupting fungal membranes, Bacillomycin D has been shown to interfere with intracellular signaling pathways by inhibiting calcium ion homeostasis within the fungal cell. By disrupting calcium signaling, Bacillomycin D induces oxidative stress, mitochondrial dysfunction, and apoptosis in fungal cells. This multifaceted mechanism of action makes Bacillomycin D effective against a variety of pathogenic fungi, including *Candida albicans* and *Aspergillus flavus* [38].

2.3.4 Inhibition of fungal biofilm formation

Biofilm protective structures are formed by fungi that make them more resistant to antifungal agents. Some B. *subtilis* peptides have the ability to prevent the formation of biofilms or disrupt pre-formed biofilms, making fungal cells more susceptible to antifungal treatments [49]. Plipastatin, a cyclic lipopeptide from *B. subtilis*, has been found to inhibit fungal biofilm formation by interfering with the initial adhesion of fungal cells to surfaces. In addition to preventing biofilm formation, plipastatin can also disrupt mature biofilms by destabilizing the fungal cell membrane and cell wall within the biofilm matrix. This antifungal activity is particularly valuable in healthcare settings where biofilm-associated infections are difficult to treat [50].

2.3.5 Disruption of mitochondrial function and induction of apoptosis

Some antifungal peptides target the mitochondria of fungal cells, leading to mitochondrial dysfunction and the induction of programmed cell death (apoptosis). This mechanism is particularly important for peptides that act intracellularly after penetrating the fungal cell membrane. For example, surfactin, produced by *B.subtilis,* is known for its ability to induce oxidative stress in fungal cells by targeting mitochondrial function. Surfactin disrupts the mitochondrial membrane potential, leading to the generation of reactive oxygen species (ROS). This oxidative stress triggers apoptotic pathways, resulting in fungal cell death. Surfactin's ability to induce apoptosis in fungal cells is particularly effective against fungal pathogens like *Candida albicans* and *Aspergillus* species [6, 51].

2.4 Antiviral peptides from *B. subtilis*

Antiviral peptides (AVPs) derived from *B. subtilis* have shown significant potential in inhibiting a wide range of viral infections. These peptides act through various molecular mechanisms, including direct interaction with viral particles, inhibition of viral entry and replication, disruption of host cell membranes, and modulation of the host immune response. The multifaceted nature of these mechanisms provides an effective antiviral defense and makes *B. subtilis*-derived AVPs a promising avenue for developing antiviral therapeutics. For example, surfactin, a cyclic lipopeptide antibiotic and biosurfactant produced by *B. subtilis*, has been shown to act as a membrane fusion inhibitor, exhibiting activity against enveloped RNA viruses like transmissible gastroenteritis virus. This prevents these viruses from entering intestinal epithelial cells. Additionally, a peptide produced by *B. subtilis* strain 3 demonstrated complete inhibition of the influenza virus in vitro, showing effectiveness comparable to oseltamivir phosphate [52]. However, it remains uncertain whether the secondary metabolites of *B. subtilis* can block infections caused by DNA viruses.

Another finding reports the antiviral properties of *B. subtilis* against a DNA virus, pseudorabies virus (PRV), that severely affects swine. Researchers isolated two strains of *B. subtilis* (L2 and V11) from broiler chicken fecal samples and evaluated their antiviral effectiveness. Notably, *B. subtilis* L2 exhibited strong antiviral activity, significantly inhibiting PRV replication in PK-15 cells. Additionally, when the metabolites of *B. subtilis* L2 were administered orally to mice, they conferred protection against lethal PRV infection, reducing viral loads in key organs such as the brain and lungs. These results highlight the potential of *B. subtilis* metabolites as antiviral agents, broadening their known antimicrobial uses and offering promising therapeutic options for PRV infections [53]. *B. subtilis* L2 has shown strong antiviral activity against PRV infection at various stages of the virus life cycle in vitro. Notably, its metabolites are more effective at inhibiting the binding of PRV compared to their effects on viral entry and replication. This suggests that these metabolites significantly block the interaction between the PRV envelope protein gC and the host cell's heparan sulfate proteoglycans. Similarly, other strains like *B. subtilis* 168 and OKB105 have been reported to prevent viral attachment by competing for viral entry receptors, such as those used by the transmissible gastroenteritis virus to infect intestinal epithelial cells [53, 54].

3. Immunomodulatory effects of *B. subtilis*

3.1 Role of *B. subtilis* peptides in modulating the immune response

B. subtilis, a probiotic species, has been recognized by the FDA as safe and is usually included in functional feed additives due to its robust probiotic properties and the convenience of its isolation and culture. The Gram-positive bacterium *B. subtilis* is well-known for its capacity to generate a wide variety of peptides with important immunomodulatory qualities to affect the immune system. Recent research showed that recombinant *B. subtilis* could elicit unique immune responses. Numerous immune cells, such as dendritic cells (DCs), macrophages, natural killer (NK) cells, and T and B cells, have been demonstrated to be directly affected by peptides produced by *B. subtilis* (**Figure 2**). They govern the release of cytokines and chemokines, produce metabolites that affect immunological responses, and regulate the activity of immune cells by interacting with cell surface receptors. There is evidence that certain AMPs of *B. subtilis* have anti-inflammatory properties in immune cells, including mast cells, neutrophils, eosinophils, macrophages, monocytes, lymphocytes, and dendritic cells. So B. *subtilis* peptides can evoke both innate and adaptive immunity.

A glycosylated AMP known as sublancin was extracted from *B. subtilis* 168. By stimulating the production of IL-1β, IL-6, and TNF-α. Sublancin affects innate immunity and improves phagocytosis, as well as the ability of methicillin-resistant *S. aureus* to induce cell death. Additionally, *B. subtilis* is used to extract macrolactin and surfactin. LPS-induced macrophages' synthesis and expression of iNOS, COX-2, and IL-6 are inhibited by macrolaction. Surfactin can hinder macrophages' ability to deliver antigens by preventing the activation of the NF-κB, p38, JNK, and Akt signaling pathways as well as the production of MHC-II and co-stimulatory molecules. Surfactin has the ability to trigger DCs to release TNF-α and IL-6, activate NF-κB signaling pathways, encourage DC maturation, and promote DC proliferative capacity [55].

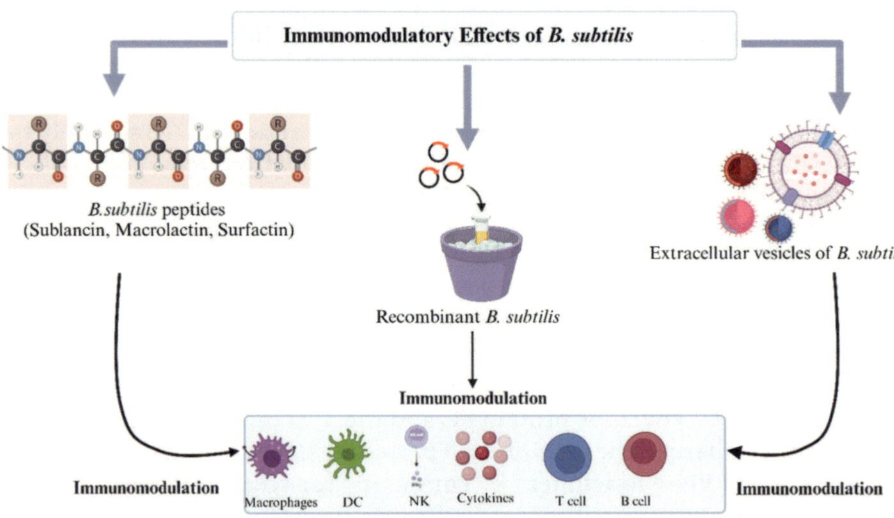

Figure 2.
Immunomodulatory effect of bioactive peptides produced by B. subtilis.

3.2 Role of recombinant *B. subtilis* in modulating the immune response

In order to evaluate the recombinant *B. subtilis* immunogenic activity, a shortened HN antigen fragment was incorporated into the surface of its spores (called *B. subtilis* RH). The findings demonstrated that the recombinant *B. subtilis* RH produced strong humoral and mucosal immune responses in mice. By promoting the growth of immune organs and increasing the number of lymphocytes in the small intestinal villi, *B. subtilis* showed potential mucosal immune adjuvant capabilities. The relative expression of inflammatory cytokines, including IL-1ß, IL-6, IL-10, TNF-a, and IFN-, in the small intestine mucosa was dramatically increased by *B. subtilis*. Moreover, *B. subtilis* demonstrated potential mucosal immunogenic properties. It provides a novel preventive approach for the chicken industry against various diseases and has the potential to be a candidate for an anti-NDV mucosal subunit vaccine [56].

3.3 Role of extracellular vesicles (EVs) of *B. subtilis* in modulating the immune response

Extracellular vesicles (EVs) are membrane-enclosed vesicles generated from cells that are used to transport bioactive substances. Outer membrane vesicles (OMVs) are a type of extracellular vesicles (EVs) that are formed by various bacteria. They have been thoroughly studied for their potential as adjuvants, immunotherapeutic agents, or vaccinations in mammals.

Using splenic leukocytes and the rainbow trout intestinal epithelial cell line (RTgutGC), EVs from the Gram-positive probiotic *B. subtilis* were generated, and their immunomodulatory potential was investigated. In both RTgutGC cells and splenocytes, *B. subtilis* EVs markedly up-regulated the transcription of a number of pro-inflammatory and antimicrobial genes. In the latter, they also up-regulated an extensive number of genes linked to B cell proliferation. In agreement, *B. subtilis* EVs improved the MHC-II surface levels and antigen-processing abilities of splenic IgM+ B cells, besides increasing the number of IgM-secreting cells in splenocyte formulations [57].

3.4 Potential applications in treating immune-related conditions

As a result of the rapid development of DNA recombination technology, *B. subtilis* has been investigated as a suitable vaccine expression vector to treat and prevent a wide range of diseases caused by bacteria, viruses, and parasites because of its ability to potentially incite the body's immune system. In order to efficiently elicit an immunological response in animals, *B. subtilis* functions as a vaccine carrier and can immunize them through the nasal cavity, sublingual, oral, and other routes. *B. subtilis* spores provide the following benefits as a live carrier of oral antigens: They are more resistant to the acidic or basic environment of the GI tract and can regulate gene expression. Lastly, they germinate first and live the longest among phagocytes [58]. *B. subtilis* is gaining significant interest as a vaccine carrier for the prevention of bacterial, viral, and parasitic illnesses for its exceptional immunological qualities. Recombinant B. *subtilis* expresses the M2 protein of influenza A, the HA protein of the highly pathogenic H5N1 avian influenza virus, the COE protein of the Porcine Epidemic Diarrhea Virus (PEDV), and the GC and GD glycoproteins of the pseudorabies virus (PRV). Furthermore, *B. subtilis* has been utilized as a vector for the expression of the FMDV (foot-and-mouth disease virus) proteins VP1 and 3A [59].

4. Application of *B. subtilis* as a vaccine carrier

In addition, it has been demonstrated that *B. subtilis* spores function as particulate vaccine adjuvants, increasing antibody responses when co-administered with antigens that are either adsorbed or admixed onto their surface (**Table 1**). In both the BALB/c and C57BL/6 mouse models, parenteral coadministration of live and dead *B. subtilis* spores can safely produce an increase in the specific antibody and T cell response to HIV gag p24 antigen. Furthermore, through the TLR2 and MyD88 signaling pathways, the spores induced DCs to produce co-stimulatory molecules and pro-inflammatory cytokines [63]. A significant obstacle in the development of a successful mucosal vaccine is identifying a suitable adjuvant. It has been demonstrated that *B. subtilis* endospores can assist in overcoming these challenges by providing a vehicle for the delivery of adjuvants and antigens. Successful development and production of recombinant spores with an adjuvant/antigen chimeric protein has been accomplished, using a piece of the *Clostridium difficile* flagellar cap FliD protein as antigen and the VQGEESNDK peptide, a fragment of human IL-1β, as an adjuvant. The obtained data demonstrate that both characteristics are exhibited by recombinant spores that provide an adjuvant/antigen chimeric protein during mouse mucosal immunization. Furthermore, the IL-1β fragment may be a useful adjuvant in mucosal vaccines based on *B. subtilis* spores [59].

5. Challenges and solutions in ensuring bioavailability and stability in the human body

Two inherent limitations of therapeutic peptide membrane impermeability along with poor in vivo stability represent significant obstacles to the development

Target pathogen	Antigen protein	Immune route	References
Virus	Capsid protein	Oral	[60]
PCV2	Collagenase equivalent		
PEDV	domain protein		
TGEV	Spike protein		
PRV	gC protein, gD protein		
HPAIV	HA protein		
FMDV	M2 protein		
	VP1 protein,		
	3A protein		
Bacteria	Sip protein	Oral	[61]
Streptococcus agalactiae	FilD protein	Oral	
Clostridium difficile	OmpC	Oral	
Salmonella	UreB protein	Oral	
Helicobacter pylori	Truncated protein 21	Nasal Intranasal	
Mycoplasma tuberculosis	P97R1, P46 protein	Mucosal	
Mycoplasma hyopneumoniae			
Parasitic	CsPmy protein	Intraperitoneal,	[62]
Clonorchis sinensis	Cysteine protease	Intragastric	
Echinococcosis granulosus	EgTrp, EgA31 protein	Oral	
Plasmodium falciparum (r*Pf*CSP)	CSP protein	Oral	
		Nasal	

Table 1.
Vaccine delivery where B. subtilis *is used as a carrier.*

of peptide drugs. The majority of *B. subtilis* peptides utilized as medicinal agents are administered intravenously rather than orally due to a number of factors. It is proven that the gastrointestinal environment has an impact on the drug's permeability across mucosal barriers, stability, and solubility. Peptides nature further limits their utility as antimicrobial agents because of their limited bioavailability and solubility, susceptibility to protease degradation, and possible toxicity and immunogenicity. But there are a few benefits to using the oral route, including its ease of usage, non-invasiveness, and self-administration convenience. To reduce the negative effects of oral administration, novel drug delivery systems (DDSs) must be developed. Developing novel drug delivery systems (DDSs) offers a promising chance to shield *B. subtilis* peptides from enzymatic and chemical destruction in the gastrointestinal tract and enhance intestinal permeability, which would result in high bioavailability [64].

6. Peptide delivery mechanisms

6.1 Biomaterial systems

Several delivery methods have been studied for *B. subtilis* peptides (**Figure 3**). Various drug delivery systems and biomaterials, such as polymer hydrogels or polar lipid assemblies, as well as less commonly used materials in pharmaceutical formulation development, like various organic nanomaterials, provide ways to regulate peptide exposure and release, protect incorporated peptides from degradation, and lessen unfavorable peptide-related side effects. Microgels and associated polymeric systems present especially intriguing alternatives. Furthermore, a wide variety of inorganic nanoparticles interact with external fields, including light and fluctuating magnetic

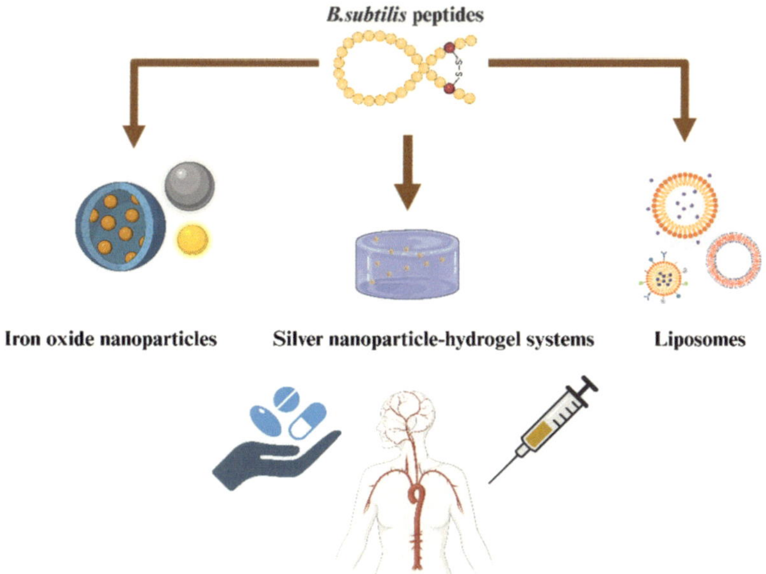

Figure 3.
Delivery systems used for bioactive peptides.

fields, creating opportunities for simultaneous diagnosis of treatment outcomes in therapeutic techniques and remotely activating the release of AMP from such delivery devices. Iron oxide nanoparticles seem especially promising in this context. Some systems, like mesoporous silicon canan nanoparticles, provide opportunities for the co-delivery of *B. subtilis* AMPs and low-MW drugs like conventional antibiotics.

An important class of biomaterials for the prevention and treatment of infections are antimicrobial nanoparticle-hydrogel systems, which are composed of antimicrobial agents (antibiotics, biological extracts, and antimicrobial peptides) loaded nanoparticles or antimicrobial nanoparticles (metal or metal oxide). Because AgNPs have an excellent dispersion capability within the hydrogel network, researchers have produced an AgNPs-loaded hydrogel made of poly (acrylamide-co-styrene sulfonic acid sodium salt) and chitosan to battle the most sensitive strains of *B. subtilis* [65].

6.2 Liposome systems

Liposomes are vesicle bilayers composed of natural phospholipids and cholesterol with an aqueous core. Liposomal delivery systems have the potential to encapsulate AMPs that are soluble in water or fat; they can also be tailored to improve drug targeting, extend the duration of the drug's action, and increase drug stability. Additionally, liposomes can help overcome multidrug resistance and minimize adverse drug reactions. The adaptability of this drug delivery system (DDS) is demonstrated by the range of *B. subtilis* AMPs that have been encapsulated into liposomes, including colistin, vancomycin, LL-37, indolicin, and polymyxin B. These AMPs can be delivered into cells by liposomes, mostly by endocytosis or adsorption. Because liposomes have a greater ability to penetrate tissues and target intracellular infections, they are a great option for encapsulating AMPs. Treatment of intracellular infections as well as oral, systemic, pulmonary, and topical administration have all been investigated for liposomes [66].

7. Preclinical and clinical studies on the safety profile and toxicity evaluation of *B. subtilis* peptides

Preclinical investigations were conducted to investigate the safety of *B. subtilis*. This genome was searched for genes encoding recognized Bacillus toxins, secondary metabolites, virulence factors, and antibiotic resistance using in silico analysis. Evaluated how *B. subtilis* lysates affected the permeability and viability of human intestinal epithelial cells (Caco-2) in culture. It was discovered that there are no known Bacillus toxins encoded in the genome. Numerous gene clusters involved in the manufacture of secondary metabolites are present in the *B. subtilis* genome; however, many of these antimicrobial compounds, such as fengycin, are shared by Bacillus species and may even have health advantages linked to the health of the gut microbiota. According to the findings of in vitro and in silico tests, *B. subtilis* is thought to be safe for ingestion by humans [67]. In another study, *B. subtilis* safety was assessed using phenotypic and genomic methods. Based on the in silico genome inquiry and cell cytotoxicity examination, BS IDCC1101 did not show any significant safety concerns, including human toxicity, antibiotic resistance transfer, or disruption to the gut microbes. Furthermore, phenotypic tests revealed that the strain did not generate any harmful compounds. Moreover, without raising any safety issues, BS IDCC1101 showed increased enzyme activity and carbohydrate utilization. In female rats, BS IDCC1101 did not exhibit acute oral toxicity. Gram-positive bacterial infections may be treated with bacitracin, a naturally occurring cyclic AMP produced from *B. subtilis*, which is being studied in several ongoing Phase IV clinical trials to evaluate the effectiveness of bacitracin in the treatment of patients with small burns, wound healing, skin infections, and surgical site infections. It's commonly used with neomycin, polymyxin B, collagenase, and honey of the medical kind. However, a trial assessing the use of bacitracin in midfacial fracture surgery was closed in April 2020 due to bacitracin toxicity [68].

8. Current limitations in the development and clinical application of *B. subtilis* AMPs

The negative characteristics of *B. subtilis* AMPs, which hinder their clinical development, include systemic toxicity, quick renal clearance, short half-lives, and sensitivity to protease breakdown. The limited bioavailability is one of the primary drawbacks of using AMPs in clinical settings. These compounds generally exhibit poor absorption at the site of action because of their difficulties in crossing biological membranes, such as the blood–brain barrier, intestinal mucosa, and cell membrane. Thus, topical, intravenous, intramuscular, or subcutaneous delivery is the most widely used. In addition to lowering absorption and bioavailability, chemical processes such as hydrolysis by stomach acid or digestive enzymes also occur. Another major barrier is its rapid elimination from the blood by high renal and hepatic clearance. The clinical application's limited selectivity is still another problem. These compounds' poor target selectivity is typically linked to cytotoxicity, which has the potential to produce hemolytic action. Additionally, there is a chance of adverse immunogenic effects due to interactions with various targets or receptors. The high development and production costs, decreased efficacy in therapeutically relevant situations, and the unanticipated rise of bacterial resistance are just a few of the obstacles facing the development of AMPs for clinical application. Although AMPs primarily affect membranes, they may also be harmful to eukaryotic cells and are not entirely specific to microbial cells [68].

9. Future research areas and potential technological advancements to overcome these challenges

It has been claimed that *B. subtilis* AMP pharmacokinetics can be enhanced by chemical modifications and administration methods. A peptide's biological activity is greatly influenced by its amino acid sequence, location, and configuration since structure and activity are interrelated. A number of chemical changes could enhance specific characteristics (such as permeability and antibacterial activity), making the AMP more stable and hence more appropriate for in vivo application. These chemical modifications include PEGylation, Lipidation, Cyclization, D-amino acids, and branched peptides (**Figure 4**).

AMP stability, bioavailability, and toxicity are reduced by utilizing strategies such as cyclization design, N- and C-terminal alterations, and the addition of the D-amino acid configuration. Enhancing AMP's biological qualities is another application for AMP nanoencapsulation. Lipid NPs, metal NPs, and polymeric nanosystems can shield the enclosed peptide against toxicity and deterioration. They can also increase efficacy and lessen negative effects.

All of these approaches could be employed in the upcoming decades to create more powerful and "individualized" medications for every patient, lowering side

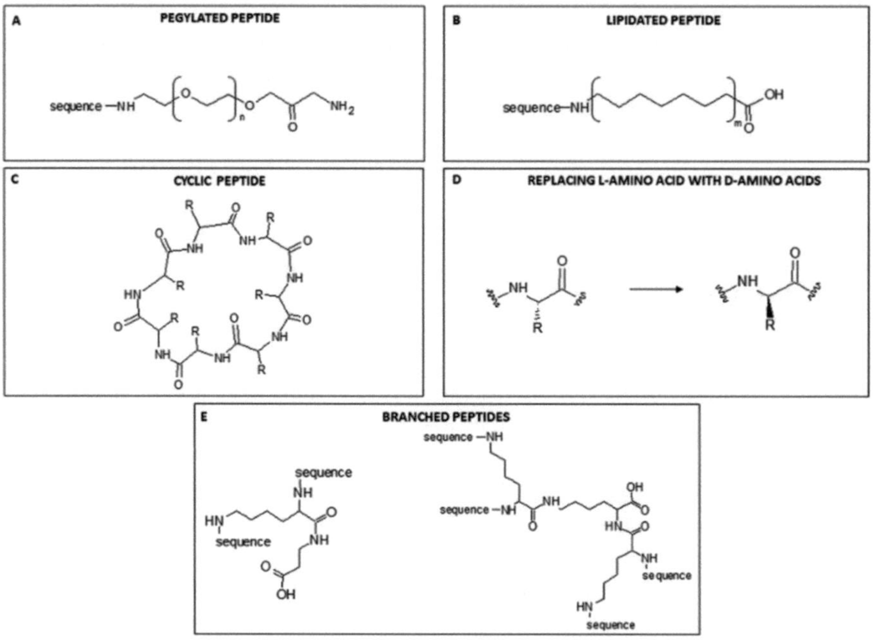

Figure 4.
Molecular structure of various peptides produced by B. subtilis.

effects and increasing efficacy. In vitro tests of nanoparticle-based AMP therapies and coatings have demonstrated encouraging outcomes, supporting the delivery of AMPs into cells for the treatment of intracellular infections as well as through bacterial biofilms and in close proximity. At this point, AMP molecule compositions are being developed for safe and efficient application, and a new phase of study is beginning. To put it another way, following a protracted era of AMP discovery and research, the emphasis is now on their druggability by enhancing and modifying delivery methods [68]. Various approaches have been devised to decrease manufacturing costs and cytotoxic consequences while enhancing the bioavailability and effectiveness of AMPs. While some companies are pursuing truncated or short AMPs in an attempt to lower production costs, it is more typical to design a delivery mechanism and provide chemical modifications in order to increase the AMPs' bioavailability and in vivo efficacy. In addition to potentially increasing efficacy, STAMPS, combination therapy with traditional antibiotics, and the choice of a counter ion at the very end of peptide synthesis may also lessen the harmful effects of AMPs [69].

10. Analysis of real-world applications and outcomes of bioactive *B.Subtilis* peptides

Phase IV clinical trials were being conducted to treat Gram-positive bacterial infections using bacitracin, a naturally occurring cyclic AMP from *B. subtilis*. The clinical study of bacitracin as a drug was successfully done to diagnose allergic contact dermatitis; the study sought to determine the appropriate concentration of the bacitracin patch. Individuals who were 18 years of age or older and had tested positive for bacitracin patch within the previous five years were considered subjects. Mekos Laboratories

AS carried out the study, which addressed a number of pertinent MeSH terms, including bacitracin, allergic contact dermatitis, patch testing, associated skin illnesses, and hypersensitivity conditions. Another clinical study of bacitracin was completed to examine the effects of time to clot and infection rate when applying bacitracin and tranexamic acid to the bleeding site following the removal of the hemodialysis fistula needle. Topical Tranexamic Acid 5% with bacitracin and Topical Tranexamic Acid 25% with bacitracin were used as a drug on 18 years and older (Adult, Older Adult) dialysis patients with fistulas (native arteriovenous). Following dialysis, each participant's arteriovenous fistula's clotting time was assessed using either 5% or 25% tranexamic acid, and the results were compared to the AV fistula's regular clotting time without the use of tranexamic acid, concluding the clotting time is 13% [70].

The lipopeptides surfactin, fengycin, and iturin, which are generated by *B. subtilis*, are utilized as biopesticides because of their potent antifungal characteristics. By preventing the growth of dangerous fungi like *Fusarium oxysporum* and *Botrytis cinerea*, they aid in crop protection. By reducing the need for chemical pesticides, the application of these peptides promotes sustainable agriculture [71].

Bacitracin and other peptides produced by *B. subtilis* are employed as antibiotics in medicinal procedures. Topical ointments containing bacitracin are frequently used to treat minor burns, wounds, and cuts and to prevent infection. The antibacterial qualities of *B. subtilis* peptides, such as subtilin and nisin, are used to preserve food. These peptides work by preventing the growth of pathogens and bacteria that cause spoilage, thus extending the shelf life of food products. Proteases and amylases are two important commercial enzymes that are derived from *B. subtilis*. These enzymes can be stabilized by the peptides created during fermentation operations, increasing their effectiveness and lowering their cost for industrial usage [72].

11. Role of modern artificial intelligence (AI) in drug design derived from *B. subtilis* peptides

Peptides exhibit a variety of biological activities that make them attractive candidates for therapeutic uses. These activities include hormone signaling, antitumor, and antibacterial properties. Therapeutic peptides have benefits but also drawbacks, like a short half-life, poor oral bioavailability, and plasma degradation susceptibility. The emergence of artificial intelligence (AI) and computational tools in peptide research has prompted the creation of sophisticated databases and procedures essential to investigating these intricate macromolecules. The incorporation of AI into peptide creation, including classifier techniques, prediction systems, and cutting-edge design made possible by deep-generative models such as variational autoencoders and generative adversarial networks.

Machine learning (ML) is a branch of artificial intelligence that focuses on statistical models and algorithms. The theory behind ML is that computers can analyze and learn from patterns in data and then use that information to solve problems, make predictions, or classify objects. Creating prediction models for peptides using ML procedures and protein sequences or structures involves four key steps: gathering and processing datasets, using numerical representation techniques, training and validating predictive models, and assessing results using traditional metrics. Depending on the goal of the prediction model, many sources may be used to get protein sequences or structures throughout the collection phase. To gather AMPs, generic databases such as LAMP2 or Peptipedia SATPdb are typically utilized. On the other hand, particular data is gathered using specialist databases such as bacteriocin peptides and anti-angiogenic peptide predictors, which are used for quorum sensing signaling peptides.

Classification models have been put into practice for medicinal purposes, such as the identification of CPPs, anticancer peptides, and anti-inflammatory peptides. Combining machine learning techniques with biomedical datasets can help find new therapeutic targets and make it easier to research biological activities, protein interactions, molecular properties, and side effects. A variety of prediction models have been used to aid in the drug discovery process, such as the Bayesian machine learning strategy BANDIT and the deep learning approach DeepDTnet, which uses phenotypic, genetic, chemical, and cellular network profiles to inform the drug development process [72].

12. Conclusion

B. subtilis peptides hold immense clinical and therapeutic potential due to their broad spectrum of activities, unique mechanisms of action, and versatility in various therapeutic applications. These peptides, including well-known examples like surfactin, fengycin, and iturin, act primarily through membrane disruption, causing cell lysis in target pathogens. This distinct mechanism minimizes the likelihood of resistance development, positioning them as promising alternatives to traditional antibiotics, particularly in the face of rising antimicrobial resistance. Beyond their antimicrobial efficacy, *B. subtilis* peptides exhibit significant potential in other therapeutic areas, such as antiviral, antifungal, antiparasitic, and anticancer treatments. Their ability to selectively target pathogens and cancer cells while sparing healthy cells broadens their therapeutic scope, making them candidates for diverse clinical applications, including wound healing and immunomodulation. Advances in peptide delivery systems, including encapsulation in nanoparticles or liposomes, have enhanced the stability, bioavailability, and targeted delivery of these peptides, addressing some of the limitations that hinder their therapeutic use, such as rapid degradation and poor solubility. Furthermore, preclinical and clinical studies have demonstrated a favorable safety profile for *B. subtilis* peptides, with low toxicity and good biocompatibility. These properties are essential for transitioning from laboratory research to clinical application. However, despite these promising characteristics, challenges remain, including optimizing peptide stability under physiological conditions and scaling up production for therapeutic use. In brief, *B. subtilis* peptides represent a valuable source of bioactive molecules with diverse therapeutic applications. Ongoing research and technological advancements in peptide delivery and stabilization will be crucial in unlocking their full clinical potential, offering new hope in the fight against infectious diseases and cancer.

Acknowledgements

The authors acknowledge the use of Grammarly for language polishing of the manuscript.

Conflict of interest

The authors declared no conflict of interest.

Author details

Sajid Iqbal[1,2]*, Mehwish Malik[2], Bushra Mustafa[2] and Hussnain Ahmed Janjua[2]

1 Oujiang Lab (Zheijiang Lab for Regenerative Medicin, Vision and Brain Health), Wenzhou, China

2 Atta-ur-Rahman School of Applied Biosciences (ASAB), National University of Sciences and Technology (NUST), Islamabad, Pakistan

*Address all correspondence to: sajidiqbalmb44@yahoo.com

References

[1] Iqbal S, Begum F, Rabaan AA, Aljeldah M, Al Shammari BR, Alawfi A, et al. Classification and multifaceted potential of secondary metabolites produced by *Bacillus subtilis* group: A comprehensive review. Molecules. 2023;**28**:927-956

[2] Hancock REW, Haney EF, Gill EE. The immunology of host defence peptides: Beyond antimicrobial activity. Nature Reviews Immunology. 2016;**16**:1-3

[3] Amber Dance. Five Ways Science Is Tackling the Antibiotic Resistance Crisis. Available from: https://www.nature.com/articles/d41586-024-02601-4

[4] Zhang QY, Bin YZ, Meng YM, Hong XY, Shao G, Ma JJ, et al. Antimicrobial peptides: Mechanism of action, activity and clinical potential. Military Medical Research. 2021;**8**:1-3

[5] Zaky AA, Simal-Gandara J, Eun JB, Shim JH, Abd El-Aty AM. Bioactivities, applications, safety, and health benefits of bioactive peptides from food and by-products: A review. Frontiers in Nutrition. 2022;**8**(3):5

[6] Kanaujia KA, Mishra N, Rajinikanth PS, Saraf SA. Antimicrobial peptides as antimicrobials for wound care management: A comprehensive review. Journal of Drug Delivery Science and Technology. 2024;**95**:1-6

[7] Nasseri S, Sharifi M. Therapeutic potential of antimicrobial peptides for wound healing. International Journal of Peptide Research and Therapeutics. 2022;**28**:1-4

[8] Nhàn NTT, Yamada T, Yamada KH. Peptide-based agents for cancer treatment: Current applications and future directions. International Journal of Molecular Sciences. 2023;**24**:1-2

[9] Chinnadurai RK, Khan N, Meghwanshi GK, Ponne S, Althobiti M, Kumar R. Current research status of anti-cancer peptides: Mechanism of action, production, and clinical applications. Biomedicine and Pharmacotherapy. 2023;**164**

[10] Chiangjong W, Chutipongtanate S, Hongeng S. Anticancer peptide: Physicochemical property, functional aspect and trend in clinical application (review). International Journal of Oncology. 2020;**57**:4-9

[11] Su Y, Liu C, Fang H, Zhang D. *Bacillus subtilis*: A universal cell factory for industry, agriculture, biomaterials and medicine. Microbial Cell Factories. 2020;**19**:1-2

[12] Pálffy R, Gardlík R, Behuliak M, Kadasi L, Turna J, Celec P. On the physiology and pathophysiology of antimicrobial peptides. Molecular Medicine. 2009;**15**:51-59

[13] Scott RW, DeGrado WF, Tew GN. De novo designed synthetic mimics of antimicrobial peptides. Current Opinion in Biotechnology. 2008;**19**:2-3

[14] Caulier S, Nannan C, Gillis A, Licciardi F, Bragard C, Mahillon J. Overview of the antimicrobial compounds produced by members of the *Bacillus subtilis* group. Frontiers in Microbiology. 2019;**10**:1-7

[15] Ongena M, Jacques P. Bacillus lipopeptides: Versatile weapons for plant disease biocontrol. Trends in Microbiology. 2008;**16**:115-125

[16] Zhao H, Yan L, Xu X, Jiang C, Shi J, Zhang Y, et al. Potential of *Bacillus subtilis* lipopeptides in anti-cancer I: Induction of apoptosis and paraptosis and inhibition of autophagy in K562 cells. AMB Express. 2018;**8**(1):1-3

[17] Gaspar D, Salomé Veiga A, Castanho MARB. From antimicrobial to anticancer peptides. A review. Frontiers in Microbiology. 2013;**4**:1-12

[18] Lin L, Chi J, Yan Y, Luo R, Feng X, Zheng Y, et al. Membrane-disruptive peptides/peptidomimetics-based therapeutics: Promising systems to combat bacteria and cancer in the drug-resistant era. Acta Pharmaceutica Sinica B. 2021;**11**:1-5

[19] Peypoux F, Bonmatin JM, Wallach J. Recent trends in the biochemistry of surfactin. Applied Microbiology and Biotechnology. 1999;**51**(5):1

[20] Wu YS, Ngai SC, Goh BH, Chan KG, Lee LH, Chuah LH. Anticancer activities of surfactin potential application of nanotechnology assisted surfactin delivery. Frontiers in Pharmacology. 2017;**8**:3-17

[21] Zakharova AA, Efimova SS, Malev VV, Ostroumova OS. Fengycin induces ion channels in lipid bilayers mimicking target fungal cell membranes. Scientific Reports. 2019;**9**(1):1

[22] Vanittanakom N, Loeffler W, Koch U, Jung G. Fengycin-a novel antifungal Lipopeptide antibiotic produced by *Bacillus subtilis* F-29-3. Journal of Antibiotics. 1986;**39**(7-10)

[23] Zhao H, Yan L, Guo L, Sun H, Huang Q, Shao D, et al. Effects of *Bacillus subtilis* iturin a on HepG2 cells in vitro and vivo. AMB Express. 2021;**11**(1):1-2

[24] Zhao H, Zhao X, Lei S, Zhang Y, Shao D, Jiang C, et al. Effect of cell culture models on the evaluation of anticancer activity and mechanism analysis of the potential bioactive compound, iturin a, produced by: *Bacillus subtilis*. Food & Function. 2019;**10**(3):3-549

[25] Fulda S. Targeting apoptosis signaling pathways for anticancer therapy. Frontiers in Oncology. 2011;**1**:1-5

[26] Leclère V, Béchet M, Adam A, Guez JS, Wathelet B, Ongena M, et al. Mycosubtilin overproduction by *Bacillus subtilis* BBG100 enhances the organism's antagonistic and biocontrol activities. Applied and Environmental Microbiology. 2005;**71**(8):1-7

[27] Lin R, Zhang Q, Yin L, Zhang Y, Yang Q, Liu K, et al. Isolation and characterization of a mycosubtilin homologue antagonizing verticillium dahliae produced by *Bacillus subtilis* strain Z15. PLoS One. 2022;**17**:19-22

[28] Yayan J, Franke KJ, Berger M, Windisch W, Rasche K. Adhesion, metastasis, and inhibition of cancer cells: A comprehensive review. Molecular Biology Reports. 2024;**51**:1

[29] Chen X et al. Bacillomycin D from *Bacillus subtilis* inhibits the invasion and migration of cancer cells via downregulation of MMP-2 and MMP-9. Journal of Applied Microbiology. 2021;**131**(4):2125-2135

[30] Lin F, Yang J, Muhammad U, Sun J, Huang Z, Li W, et al. Bacillomycin D-C16 triggers apoptosis of gastric cancer cells through the PI3K/Akt and FoxO3a signaling pathways. Anti-Cancer Drugs. 2019;**30**(1):1-4

[31] Geiger C, Korn SM, Häsler M, Peetz O, Martin J, Kötter P, et al. LanI-mediated lantibiotic immunity in *Bacillus subtilis*: Functional analysis. Applied

and Environmental Microbiology. 2019;**85**(11):9-16

[32] Dan AK, Manna A, Ghosh S, Sikdar S, Sahu R, Parhi PK, et al. Molecular mechanisms of the lipopeptides from *Bacillus subtilis* in the apoptosis of cancer cells—A review on its current status in different cancer cell lines. Advances in Cancer Biology - Metastasis. 2021;**3**:4-9

[33] Yan L, Liu G, Zhao B, Pang B, Wu W, Ai C, et al. Novel biomedical functions of surfactin A from *Bacillus subtilis* in wound healing promotion and scar inhibition. Journal of Agricultural and Food Chemistry. 2020;**68**(26):5-6

[34] Arima K et al. Surfactin inhibits VEGF-induced angiogenesis by reducing the VEGF receptor expression. Journal of Cellular Physiology. 2010;**2010**:1-9

[35] Chen X, Lu Y, Shan M, Zhao H, Lu Z, Lu Y. A mini-review: Mechanism of antimicrobial action and application of surfactin. World Journal of Microbiology and Biotechnology. 2022;**38**:3-6

[36] Zhao H, Shao D, Jiang C, Shi J, Li Q, Huang Q, et al. Biological activity of lipopeptides from bacillus. Applied Microbiology and Biotechnology. 2017;**101**:1-5

[37] Maget-Dana R, Peypoux F. Iturins, a special class of pore-forming lipopeptides: Biological and physicochemical properties. Toxicology. 1994;**87**(1-3):10-17

[38] Tran C, Cock IE, Chen X, Feng Y. Antimicrobial bacillus: Metabolites and their mode of action. Antibiotics. 2022;**11**:8-10

[39] Nannan C, Vu HQ, Gillis A, Caulier S, Nguyen TTT, Mahillon J. Bacilysin within the *Bacillus subtilis* group: Gene prevalence versus antagonistic activity against gram-negative foodborne pathogens. Journal of Biotechnology. 2021;**327**:2-7

[40] Islam T, Rabbee MF, Choi J, Baek KH. Biosynthesis, molecular regulation, and application of Bacilysin produced by bacillus species. Metabolites. 2022;**12**:2-5

[41] Parisot J, Carey S, Breukink E, Chan WC, Narbad A, Bonev B. Molecular mechanism of target recognition by subtilin, a class I lanthionine antibiotic. Antimicrobial Agents and Chemotherapy. 2008;**52**(2):1-7

[42] Chen M, Lin N, Liu X, Tang X, Wang Z, Zhang D. A novel antimicrobial peptide screened by a *Bacillus subtilis* expression system, derived from Larimichthys crocea ferritin H, exerting bactericidal and parasiticidal activities. Frontiers in Immunology. 2023;**14**:6-13

[43] Zhu J, Wang S, Wang C, Wang Z, Luo G, Li J, et al. Microbial synthesis of bacitracin: Recent progress, challenges, and prospects. Synthetic and Systems Biotechnology. 2023;**8**:1-3

[44] Leistikow KR, May DS, Suh WS, Vargas Asensio G, Schaenzer AJ, Currie CR, et al. *Bacillus subtilis* -derived peptides disrupt quorum sensing and biofilm assembly in multidrug-resistant *Staphylococcus aureus*. mSystems. 2024;**9**(8):3-11

[45] Raju DV, Nagarajan A, Pandit S, Nag M, Lahiri D, Upadhye V. Effect of bacterial quorum sensing and mechanism of antimicrobial resistance. Biocatalysis and Agricultural Biotechnology. 2022;**43**:1-4

[46] Peypoux F, Bonmatin JM, Wallach J. MINI-REVIEW recent trends in the biochemistry of surfactin. Applied Microbiology and Biotechnology. 1999;**51**(5):553-563

[47] Ramesh S, Roy U, Roy S, Rudramurthy SM. A promising antifungal lipopeptide from *Bacillus subtilis*: Its characterization and insight into the mode of action. Applied Microbiology and Biotechnology. 2024;**108**(1):1-18

[48] Yu C, Liu X, Zhang X, Zhang M, Gu Y, Ali Q, et al. Mycosubtilin produced by *Bacillus subtilis* ATCC6633 inhibits growth and mycotoxin biosynthesis of fusarium graminearum and fusarium verticillioides. Toxins (Basel). 2021;**13**(11):3-9

[49] Vahidinasab M, Lilge L, Reinfurt A, Pfannstiel J, Henkel M, Morabbi Heravi K, et al. Construction and description of a constitutive plipastatin mono-producing *Bacillus subtilis*. Microbial Cell Factories. 2020;**19**(1):1-5

[50] Batool M, Khalid MH, Hassan MN, Hafeez FY. Homology modeling of an antifungal metabolite plipastatin synthase from the *Bacillus subtilis* 168. Bioinformation. 2011;**7**(8):1-3

[51] Meena KR, Kanwar SS. Lipopeptides as the antifungal and antibacterial agents: Applications in food safety and therapeutics. BioMed Research International. 2015;**2015**:2-6

[52] Yuan L, Zhang S, Wang Y, Li Y, Wang X, Yang Q. Surfactin inhibits membrane fusion during invasion of epithelial cells by enveloped viruses. Journal of Virology. 2018;**92**(21):2-16

[53] Wang X, Hao G, Zhou M, Chen M, Ling H, Shang Y. Secondary metabolites of *Bacillus subtilis* L2 show antiviral activity against pseudorabies virus. Frontiers in Microbiology. 2023;**14**:7-9

[54] Wang Y, Moon A, Huang J, Sun Y, Qiu HJ. Antiviral effects and underlying mechanisms of probiotics as promising antivirals. Frontiers in Cellular and Infection Microbiology. 2022;**12**:12-25

[55] Li H, Niu J, Wang X, Niu M, Liao C. The contribution of antimicrobial peptides to immune cell function: A review of recent advances. Pharmaceutics. 2023;**15**:2-13

[56] Li J, Yang M, Chen B, Wang Z, Cao Y, Yang Y, et al. Evaluation of the immunity responses in mice to recombinant *Bacillus subtilis* displaying Newcastle disease virus HN protein truncations. Microorganisms. 2024;**12**(3):12-15

[57] Vicente-Gil S, Nuñez-Ortiz N, Morel E, Serra CR, Docando F, Díaz-Rosales P, et al. Immunomodulatory properties of *Bacillus subtilis* extracellular vesicles on rainbow trout intestinal cells and splenic leukocytes. Frontiers in Immunology. 2024;**15**:8-15

[58] Yuan C, Ji X, Zhang Y, Liu X, Ding L, Li J, et al. Important role of *Bacillus subtilis* as a probiotic and vaccine carrier in animal health maintenance. World Journal of Microbiology and Biotechnology. 2024;**40**:4-9

[59] Potocki W, Negri A, Peszyńska-Sularz G, Hinc K, Obuchowski M, Iwanicki A. IL-1 fragment modulates immune response elicited by recombinant *Bacillus subtilis* spores presenting an antigen/adjuvant chimeric protein. Molecular Biotechnology. 2018;**60**(11):810-819

[60] Lin J, Mou C, Zhang S, Zhu L, Li Y, Yang Q. Immune responses induced by recombinant *Bacillus subtilis* expressing the PEDV spike protein targeted at microfold cells. Veterinary Sciences. 2022;**9**(5):2-10

[61] Saggese A, Baccigalupi L, Donadio G, Ricca E, Isticato R. The bacterial spore

as a mucosal vaccine delivery system. International Journal of Molecular Sciences. 2023;**24**:8-13

[62] de Almeida MEM, Alves KCS, de Vasconcelos MGS, Pinto TS, Glória JC, Chaves YO, et al. *Bacillus subtilis* spores as delivery system for nasal plasmodium falciparum circumsporozoite surface protein immunization in a murine model. Scientific Reports. 2022;**12**(1):2-6

[63] De Souza RD, Batista MT, Luiz WB, Cavalcante RCM, Amorim JH, Bizerra RSP, et al. *Bacillus subtilis* spores as vaccine adjuvants: Further insights into the mechanisms of action. PLoS One. 2014;**9**(1):2-7

[64] Deshayes C, Arafath MN, Apaire-Marchais V, Roger E. Drug delivery systems for the oral administration of antimicrobial peptides: Promising tools to treat infectious diseases. Frontiers in Medical Technology. 2021;**3**:6-10

[65] Ahmad N, Bukhari SNA, Hussain MA, Ejaz H, Munir MU, Amjad MW. Nanoparticles incorporated hydrogels for delivery of antimicrobial agents: Developments and trends. RSC Advances. 2024;**14**(19):13535-13564

[66] van Gent ME, Ali M, Nibbering PH, Kłodzińska SN. Current advances in lipid and polymeric antimicrobial peptide delivery systems and coatings for the prevention and treatment of bacterial infections. Pharmaceutics. 2021;**13**:3-15

[67] Brutscher LM, Borgmeier C, Garvey SM, Spears JL. Preclinical safety assessment of *Bacillus subtilis* BS50 for probiotic and food applications. Microorganisms. 2022;**10**(5):1-14

[68] Cresti L, Cappello G, Pini A. Antimicrobial peptides towards clinical application—A long history to be concluded. International Journal of Molecular Sciences. 2024;**25**:4-13

[69] Dijksteel GS, Ulrich MMW, Middelkoop E, Boekema BKHL. Review: Lessons learned from clinical trials using antimicrobial peptides (AMPs). Frontiers in Microbiology. 2021;**12**:10-12

[70] Moretta A, Scieuzo C, Petrone AM, Salvia R, Manniello MD, Franco A, et al. Antimicrobial peptides: A new Hope in biomedical and pharmaceutical fields. Frontiers in Cellular and Infection Microbiology. 2021;**11**:6-18

[71] Iqbal S, Ullah N, Janjua HA. In vitro evaluation and genome mining of *Bacillus subtilis* strain rs10 reveals its biocontrol and plant growth-promoting potential. Agriculture (Switzerland). 2021;**11**(12):11-14

[72] Goles M, Daza A, Cabas-Mora G, Sarmiento-Varón L, Sepúlveda-Yañez J, Anvari-Kazemabad H, et al. Peptide-based drug discovery through artificial intelligence: Towards an autonomous design of therapeutic peptides. Briefings in Bioinformatics. 2024;**25**:4-11

Chapter 5

Bacillus subtilis: A Biological Marvel in the Domain of Agriculture and Environmental Science

Sonam Shrirang Shinde, Viraj Vivek Gaonkar, Humaira Mushtaq Mukadam and Shikha Vikrant Gaikwad

Abstract

Bacillus subtills is a Gram-positive, rod-shaped, aerobic, non-pathogenic bacterium that synthesizes resilient endospores. Due to the capability of forming spores, the organism has ecological versatility that allows the organism to thrive in distinct environments such as soil, rhizospheric zones of plants, and even in the gastrointestinal tracts of animals. It is widely known as a plant growth-promoting rhizobacterium (PGPR) that enhances plants' growth by producing various primary and secondary metabolites such as phytohormones, volatile organic compounds (VOC), enzymes (exo), biosurfactants, siderophores, solubilizing phosphate, and fixing nitrogen. The bacterium's utility in agriculture is further supported by various formulation and delivery methods, enhancing its effectiveness as a biopesticide and biofertilizer. Additionally, *B. subtilis* contributes to soil health and sustainability by forming protective biofilms and generating antimicrobial compounds, which suppress the progression of deleterious microorganisms. Metabolites of the bacterium also degrade and remediates heavy metals and hydrocarbons that aids in maintaining sustainability in the environment. Despite its wide-ranging values, challenges are still there in terms of its usage optimization. Future perspectives are highly required that would enhance all its beneficial traits and integrate *B. subtilis* into integrated pest management (IPM) systems as a potential pollutant remediator to promote sustainable agricultural and environmental practices, which are documented in the -chapter.

Keywords: *Bacillus subtilis*, plant growth-promoting rhizobacteria (PGPR), biosurfactants, sustainable agricultural and environmental practices, integrated pest management

1. Introduction

The bacterium, *Bacillus subtilis* which is well-known as soil-dwelling prokaryote, was discovered by Christian Gottfried Ehrenberg [1]. It is a Gram-positive bacterium with rod-shaped cells, 2–6 μm in length and less than 1 μm in diameter. The organism has a single circular chromosome of 4.2 million base pairs long, encoding 4100 genes [2]. The bacterium has a single flagellated or non-flagellated cell that shows stochastic

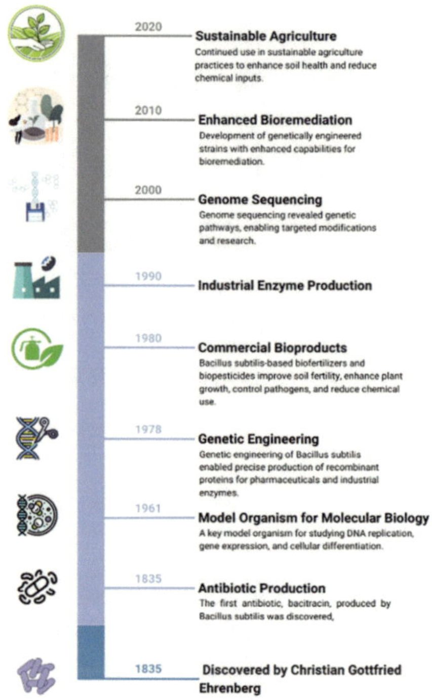

Figure 1.
Historical perspective on the use of Bacillus subtilis.

variation in the expression of motility-related genes [3] and allows the bacterium to develop a biofilm [4]. An ability to form resilient spore provides an additional advantage to the bacterium in terms of survivability under extreme conditions [5]. In recent years, *B. subtilis* is becoming a model organism for the biofilm study due to its ability to diverse phenotypes within an isogenic population [4].

In 1835, the first antibiotic was discovered from *B. subtilis* and from the year 1980 onwards, the bacterium was highlighted due to its secretion of a variety of proteins, enzymes and bioactive molecules, that is making the bacterium an important plant growth promoter and as a pollutant remediator [5]. The histological approaches of the bacterium are highlighted in **Figure 1** from the year 1835 to 2020.

2. Mechanisms of plant growth enhancement by *Bacillus subtilis*

2.1 Synthesis of phytohormones

Phytohormones such as Auxins, Cytokinins, Gibberellins, Abscisic acid, Salicylic acid, and Jasmonic acid have vital impact on the plants' growth. *B. subtilis* is reported as a secretor of these phytohormones that enhances plants' growth and yield by improving rhizobacterial colonization [6, 7] or by increasing defense mechanisms [8, 9]. *B. subtilis* is also reported to be a producer of volatile organic compounds (VOCs) like albuterol and 1,3-propanediol, that trigger gene expression for Auxin, Gibberellin, Cytokinin, and Ethylene biosynthesis [10]. Among all phytohormones, indole-3-acetic acid (IAA) is a key player in plant physiology, influencing cell division, expansion, differentiation, germination, phototropism, geotropism, and stress alleviation [11]. *B. subtilis* are also known to produce IAA [12] at significant levels. Additionally, it is the only bacterium that can produce multiple auxins such as indole-3-acetic acid (IAA), indole-3-butyric acid (IBA), and indole-3-propionic acid (IPA) [13, 14]. IAA synthesis in *B. subtilis* is reported to be increased under temperature gradients [15–17]. Additionally, IAA-producing *B. subtilis* strains is reported to improve salinity tolerance in crop [18, 19]. Cytokinins are vital for multiple facets of plant growth and development, such as embryogenesis, meristem activity, vascular formation, root lengthening, lateral root and nodule development, and apical dominance [20]. *B. subtilis* is known to produce Cytokinins up to 150 ng/mL [21–24]. Additionally, Gibberellins and Abscisic acid (ABA), are also secreted by *B. subtilis* which enhances plant tolerance to drought and salinity [25, 26].

2.2 Enhancement of nutrient availability

Plant growth can be enhanced by aiding nutrient acquisition. Plant growth-promoting rhizobacteria (PGPR) accomplish the accessibility of nutrients by fixing nitrogen and solubilizing inorganic phosphates [27].

2.2.1 Nitrogen fixation

Nitrogen is an essential component for plant development, but plants cannot absorb directly atmospheric nitrogen. To satisfy the rising food demands, farmers use large amounts of nitrogenous fertilizers, but it is impacting drastically on the functionality of macro and microorganisms [28]. Nitrogen-fixing bacteria plays a vital role in transforming nitrogen into ammonia which facilitates biological nitrogen fixation. *B. subtilis* has the ability to fix atmospheric nitrogen and native rhizobacterial colonization [29]. The bacterium has also been reported to reduce ammonia emissions by 44% and ammonia levels [30]. Sun and his coworkers [31] reported that replacing 50% of urea with *B. subtilis* biofertilizer decreased nitrogen loss by 54%.

2.2.2 Phosphate solubilization

Phosphorus is necessary for plant growth, aiding in flowering, seed formation, disease resistance, shoot strength, and root development [32]. However, plants can only access about 4% of soil phosphorus as orthophosphate [33]. It is reported by many researchers, *B. subtilis* solubilizes phosphorus even in stressful conditions [34, 35]. This highlights the bacterium's applicability to be used as a PGPR under extreme conditions [36–39].

3. *Bacillus subtilis* as a biocontrol agent for phytopathogens

3.1 Mechanisms of biocontrol

B. subtilis plays a crucial role in managing plant diseases by promoting plants' growth, inducing systemic resistance, forming biofilms, and lysing cells of deleterious phytopathogens [40]. These traits are shown by the bacterium due to the potential production of secondary metabolites, such as cell-wall-degrading enzymes, and antioxidants, that indirectly promotes plant growth [1]. The mechanisms of *B. subtilis* are defined in **Table 1**, by which it controls the growth of phytopathogens.

B. subtilis strain	Mechanism	Phytopathogen	References
BS-01	Production of VOC	*Alternaria solani*	[41]
FJ3	Nutrient acquisition, production of IAA, biofilm, hydrolytic enzyme	*Fusarium oxysporum*	[42]
FZV-1	Production of surfactin, fengycin, and siderophores	*Fusarium solani*	[43]
SR22	Secondary bioactive metabolites	*Rhizoctonia solani*	[44]
EMCCN 1211	Induction of ISR	*Potato virus Y*	[45]
V26	Production of surfactin, fengycin, iturin, bacillomycin	*Fusarium oxysporum, Fusarium solani*	[46]
SL-6	Production of surfactin, fengycin, iturin	*Alternaria alternata, Botrytis cineria*	[47]
MBI 600	Production of fengycin	*Botrytis cineria*	[48]
NCD-2	Production of surfactin, fengycin, iturin	*Rhizoctonia solani AG-8*	[49]

Table 1.
Bacillus subtilis *as a biocontrol agent.*

3.1.1 Secondary metabolites

B. subtilis is an effective biocontrol bacterium owing to its ability to produce various secondary metabolites such as biosurfactants-lipopeptides, bacteriocins, exoenzymes, and Volatile Organic Compounds (VOCs) [50]. Approximately 2428 antimicrobial peptides have been identified in *Bacillus* strains, with 4.5–15.4% of their genomes that are dedicated to synthesizing these metabolites [51]. Key cyclic lipopeptides including iturins, fengycins, and surfactins inhibit the phytopathogen by disrupting cell membranes and interfering with their cellular processes [52]. Fengycins and iturins are notable for disintegrating fungal cell membrane integrity and inhibiting spore germination [53]. It is reported that the survival rate of *Arabidopsis thaliana* increased remarkably when it was inoculated with surfactin-producing *B. subtilis*, as compared to non-surfactin-producing *B. subtilis* mutant [54]. Inoculation with surfactin-producing *B. subtilis* when associated with plant polysaccharides improves root colonization, motility, and biofilm formation [55]. *B. subtilis* also produces bacteriocins like plantazolicin and subtilin which are effective against phytopathogens growth [56, 57]. *B. subtilis* also produces exoenzymes such as proteases and chitinases that disrupt fungal cell walls [58]. Enzymatic antagonistic actions are crucial for managing fungi-induced plant diseases. Key lytic enzymes which include chitinases, cellulases, proteases, and β-1,3-glucanases that degrade pathogens' cell walls [59], are reported to be present in *B. subtilis* [60]. The scanning electron microphotographs revealed the deformations such as perforation, cell wall lysis, and cytoplasmic disintegration which highlights the applicability of the bacterium in the domain of agriculture as a biocontrol agent [61].

3.1.2 Production of siderophore

Siderophores are iron-chelating compounds synthesized by various microbes to enhance iron uptake. These siderophores are essential for plant nutrition, and stress alleviation. At the same time, they play a vital function in controlling the growth of phytopathogens [62]. *B. subtilis* is noted as a potential siderophore producer [63, 64]. It is reported that the catecholate siderophore of *B. subtilis* inhibited resistant fungus *Ralstonia solanacearum* growth and reduced disease severity by 40% [65].

3.1.3 Induction of systemic resistance in plants against pathogens

Induced Systemic Resistance (ISR) enhances plant defenses against both biotic and abiotic stressors. *B. subtilis* induces ISR by producing defense-related enzymes like peroxidase, polyphenol oxidase, and phenylalanine ammonia lyase, triggering ultrastructural and cytochemical changes in host cells during pathogen attacks [66]. *B. subtilis* strain MBI600 promoted the growth of the plant and ISR against soil-borne pathogens via salicylic acid and jasmonic acid/ethylene signaling pathways [48]. It is also reported that *B. subtilis* disrupted viral replication and upregulated pathogenesis-related genes, reducing symptoms and improving yield of the plant under infection due to *Pepper Golden Mosaic Virus* [67]. The bacterium has the capability of reprogramming the plant genome, involving RNA interference (RNAi) and microRNAs (miRNAs) [68] through which it can improve the ISR.

3.1.4 Competition for space and resources

Biological control involves competition for resources and space between pathogens and nonpathogenic organisms around a host plant. Effective root colonization relies on traits like motility, biofilm formation, and signaling interactions with the plant [58]. Root exudates attract microorganisms through bacterial chemotaxis, aiding in initial host-microbe interactions and root system colonization [69]. It is reported *B. subtilis* strains has the potential to form biofilms on plant roots, enabling long-term rhizosphere colonization and competition with pathogens [70, 71] that makes the bacterium competent biocontrol agent.

3.2 Development and commercialization of *B. subtilis*-based biocontrol agents

Chemical derived pesticides and fertilizers are in use since decades to control phytopathogens and to boost the yield of plants. On the other hand, they harm soil biodiversity, reduce soil respiration, and impart many other adverse effects on soil macroorganisms' health and development [72–74]. Microbes offer a safer alternative because of their target-specific impact and their ability to minimize bioaccumulation [75]. The Food and Drug Administration has declared *B. subtilis* a safe bacterium, which is why it is commercially available as a biocontrol agent [76]. **Table 2** mentions commercially available *B. subtilis* biocontrol agents [77].

4. Applications of *B. subtilis* in environmental remediation

4.1 Biodegradation of pollutants

The interest in using microbial functions within complex multiphase systems for bioremediation has surged due to their effectiveness, environmental friendliness, and cost efficiency. This approach addresses heavy metal contamination and hydrocarbon pollution, both of which pose significant environmental and health risks [78, 79]. The biodegradation potential of *B. subtilis* is due to its ability to produce a diverse array of

B. subtilis strain	Trade name	Target disease	Crop	Manufacturer
B246	Avogreen	Cercospora spot	Avocado	Stimulant, South Africa
NSRS89-24+ MK-007	Biobest	Sheath blight, Blast, Brown spot	Rice	AppliedChem, Thailand
AP-01	Larminar	Bacterial wilt, Damping-off, Frogeye leaf spot	Vegetable, fruit, ornamental and field crops	
MBI 600	HiStick	Fungal root disease	Field crops	Becker Underwood, USA
	Subtilex	Botrytis, Powdery mildew, Anthracnose	Field, ornamental and vegetable crops	
GB03	Kodiak	Seed and root disease	Field and vegetable crops	Bayer CropScience, USA
QST 713	Rhapsody	Powdery mildew, Fusarium root and stem rot, Pythium crown and root rot, Gummy stem blight	Ornamental, vegetable and fruit greenhouse crops	AgraQuest, USA
	Serenade	Rusts, Powdery mildews	Vegetable, wine, fruit and nut crops	
AFS032321	Theia	Bacterial disease, Fire blight, Powdery mildew	Fruit and tuber crops	AgBiome, USA
QST 713	CEASE	Botrytis, Powdery mildew, Bacterial leaf spots	Ornamental trees, fruits and vegetables grown in greenhouse	BioWorks, USA
Bacillus subtilis	Katyayani *Bacillus subtilis*	Root rot, Root wilt, Seedling rot	Fruit and vegetable crops	Katyayani, India
MCC 0067	Biotilis	Fungal diseases	Fruit, vegetable and field crops	AgriLife, India

Table 2.
Bacillus subtilis-*based commercial biocontrol agents.*

enzymes, biosurfactants, and biodegradative compounds that were in limelight from the year 2010 onwards. This intricate interplay of enzymatic and metabolic pathways allows *B. subtilis* to effectively break down complex organic contaminants, converting them into less toxic and simpler forms [1]. The capability of forming resilient spores allows the organism to survive in harsh conditions at contaminated sites and continue pollutant degradation over time [80].

4.1.1 Heavy metal detoxification

The genus *Bacillus* uses several strategies to remove heavy metals from contaminated environments such as biosorption, bioaccumulation, and bioprecipitation. Biosorption is a passive process where metal ions bind to the cell surface or extracellular polymeric substances (EPS) through interactions like ion exchange or electrostatic attraction, reducing metal mobility and bioavailability [81]. Although, in bioaccumulation, the active uptake and intracellular storage of metal ions concentrate them and reduce their environmental toxicity. In comparison with bioprecipitation, it converts dissolved metal ions into insoluble precipitates via enzymatic or metabolic processes, immobilizing them and minimizing environmental impact. These strategies enhance bioremediation efforts, with effectiveness influenced by factors like buffering capacity, organic matter, and target metal concentrations [79, 82, 83]. Ponia et al. proved that *B. subtilis* removed 88% of cadmium ions at acidic pH [84]. An engineered *B. subtilis* was able to lower the percentage of various elements at the rate of more than 95% (lead, mercury and copper) in water, and, in combination with biochar, more pronounced effects were reported for lead for the maize plant [85]. In wastewater treatment, *B. subtilis* reduced chromium levels by up to 91% [86]. *B. subtilis* as a potential candidate showed all these strategies that are making the bacterium a competent molecule for detoxification and remediation of pollutants.

4.1.2 Hydrocarbon degradation

Hydrocarbon is a major contaminant present in water and soil. Its biodegradation is a major challenge because of its low solubility in water [87]. *Bacillus* species are known to produce amphipathic molecules known as biosurfactants (BS). The molecule enhances solubility and bioavailability of these hydrocarbons by reducing surface tension and forming emulsions, improving microbial interaction and biodegradation rates for microbes [88]. Biosurfactants or biosurfactant-producing bacteria are used, particularly at oil and hydrophobic contaminant sites. Many researchers reported the presence of *B. subtilis* in the areas that are highly contaminated with hydrocarbons where they produce biosurfactants such as surfactin, iturin, and fengycin that increase the solubility of hydrocarbons. Inside *B. subtilis* specialized enzymes such as oxygenases and dehydrogenases further catalyze the oxidation of these hydrocarbons converting them into less toxic forms such as carbon dioxide and water, thus effectively reducing environmental impact of the hydrocarbon [78, 89, 90].

5. Formulation and delivery methods of *Bacillus subtilis* in agriculture

The Food and Agriculture Organization (FAO) of the United Nations estimates that pathogenic diseases account for 20–40% of losses in agricultural productivity [91]. Overusing chemically synthesized fertilizers negatively affects ecosystem function, biosphere, and the sustainability of agriculture. An essential part of Integrated Agricultural Management Systems (ICMS) is biological control, defined as using beneficial microbes to minimize the detrimental impact of phytopathogens and enhance beneficial plant responses [1]. The *Bacillus* species is a highly studied biocontrol agent that functions as a biopesticide because of its primary ability to create endospores that allows to survive in adverse conditions resiliently [51]. Microorganisms that develop endospores endures robust processing steps during large-scale manufacture, ensuring formulation resistance, stability, and effectiveness [92–94]. *Bacillus*-based microbial formulations are widely used in various other fields other than agriculture and environment such as pharmaceuticals. Different types of formulations, such as solid (granules and powder) and liquid formulations, are used with specific substances added during production like lactose monohydrate, PVP K-30, sodium alginate, talc, clay, cellulose, carboxymethyl cellulose and various oils and sugars [95]. Application methods for microbial bioformulations, includes foliar spray, root dip, soil drenching, seed treatment, and compost activation [96].

5.1 Techniques for mass production and formulation of *B. subtilis*-based products

The production process of microbial bioformulations, particularly focusing on *Bacillus* species, involves controlled cultivation conditions (oxygen transfer, agitation), selection of media, separation and purification of the product, formulation of the product, addition of the stabilizers and additives in the formulation, and quality control testing to avoid competition between cells. Producing high-quality biomass that may be readily absorbed into a formulation while maintaining the appropriate cell density and sporulation efficiency is the main objective of microbe cultivation [97]. The optimization of fermentation procedures for maximum total biomass yields as well as maximum biomass efficacy and formulation amenability is a critical first step toward maintaining biomass viability during stabilization, drying, and rehydration. Fermentation procedures should usually be created to optimize the formation of effective spores rather than vegetative cells when creating biomass of *Bacillus* spp. [98, 99]. **Figure 2** highlights the different formulations and delivery methods of *B. subtilis* in the domain of agriculture.

5.2 Application methods

5.2.1 Seed biopriming

A plant's ability to sustain the growth of the antagonist and its ability to be positioned where it is most required makes seed treatment an excellent method for introducing antagonists to control infections [100]. It has been demonstrated that seed treatments are a key factor in determining rhizosphere and rhizoplane colonization since they promote the antagonistic bacterium's early colonization of germination seedlings. It is regarded as one of the most feasible methods of distributing biological control agents [101], it presents several benefits over bulk soil treatments or in-furrow applications. Studies have demonstrated that applying *B. subtilis* to soil or seeds may efficiently protect plants from various phytopathogens [102, 103]. It was reported,

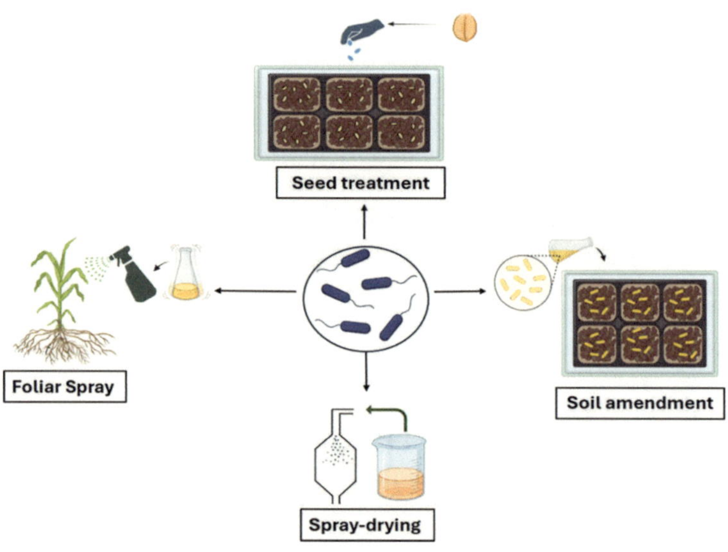

Figure 2.
Formulation and delivery methods of Bacillus subtilis *in agriculture.*

addition of *B. subtilis*, and Zimmu leaves extract when used in seed biopriming showed highest seed germination rate and significant reduction in the early blight disease [104]. On the other hand, biopriming treatments of *B. subtilis* were also reported to increase seed germination indices (percentage and velocity) under extremely saline conditions for the plant canola [105].

5.2.2 Foliar spray

A foliar spray of *B. subtilis* can make plants resist fungal diseases such as powdery mildew, down mildew, anthracnose, and leaf blight that are reported for numerous crops, such as oil seeds, cotton, tomatoes, peas, beans, millet, pulses, onions, garlic, and basil. The foliar application of the PGPB involves spraying the plant growth-promoting bacterial growth along with its metabolites. The effectiveness of *B. subtilis* strain HA1 culture filtrate with dual foliar application in shielding tomato plants against *Tobacco mosaic virus* (TMV) disease was evaluated in a greenhouse environment with significant increases in shoot and root parameters [106] and photosynthetic rate up to 89% [107]. Spray drying, fluidized bed drying, and freeze drying are some of the techniques used in formulations. Although most common method is freeze-drying, however spray drying works four to seven times better [108, 109]. The ability of *B. subtilis* to generate endospores makes it a viable option for preserving biological products after spray-drying due to its ability to withstand extreme temperatures. In the year 2012, Mendizabal and his coworkers demonstrated *B. subtills* spray-dried PA-8 formulations with an extended shelf life that continue to work to prevent *Monilinia* spp. from causing brown rot in nectarine and peach fruit [110].

5.2.3 Soil amendment

In agroecosystems, soil-beneficial microorganisms have been used for many years as an ecologically significant soil additive [111]. Soil-beneficial microorganisms mostly comprise *Bacillus* and *Pseudomonas* species, which exhibit outstanding qualities for improving soil quality [112]. *B. subtilis*, a commonly known bacterium plays a key role in enhancing the ability of plants to withstand both biotic and abiotic stresses [113]. The recent study of Charles and his coworkers highlighted, soil amendment with *B. subtilis* along with *Pseudomonas fluorescens* have impacted on nitrogen fertility variations, which are regulated by soil enzymatic activities [114].

6. Future perspectives and challenges and in the use of *B. subtilis*

B. subtilis serves as a model prokaryote with unique mechanisms and genetic pathways, that are not universally applicable to all bacterial species [115]. The successful stories of *B. subtilis* in enhancing plant growth, controlling the growth of phytopathogens, restoring contaminated habitats and advancing sustainable farming methods are well accepted. However, challenges in regulatory networks and cellular machinery complexity require further elucidation. It is highly recommended that the Synthetic Biology field should be explored by using *B. subtilis* information for tailored tasks [116], translating laboratory is having high potentiality of solving real-world problems. Although *B. subtilis* has tremendous potential across a range of industries, further research is needed to determine its efficacy and scalability in practical world contexts in other domains other than agricultural and environment.

6.1 Limitations and challenges in the field application of *B. subtilis*

Although *B. subtilis* is widely accepted for its efficiencies but still its formulation or when mixed with other microbes fail to satisfy farmers in the field, even after they have been reported successfully as biofertilizers or biocontrol during *in vitro* or *in situ* trials [117]. Thus, to widen the shelf life and field performance of *B. subtilis*, adequate storage and transportation are desired. The right management of storage and transportation minimizes the bacterial population, which leads to imbalance of field performance [118]. There are various ongoing innovations in the delivery systems for enhanced efficacy and stability of microbial bioformulations, especially those containing *Bacillus* species, such as encapsulation technologies (microencapsulation and nanoencapsulation) that protect microbial cells from environmental stresses and improve their survival rates [119, 120]. On the other hand, the utilization of biodegradable, environmentally friendly carriers and additions of adjuvants or additives can also play an imperative role for sustained release of bioformulations and maintaining their survivability in the target environment [121, 122] for a longer period of time. The application of nanotechnology to improve the penetration and uptake of bioformulations by plants, enhancing their overall efficacy [123] can again play an important role which needs uttermost attention to fulfill the demand for quality food while maintaining agroecosystems where the excessive usage of synthetic fertilizers and pesticides has harmed natural predators, soil biota, and human health, leading to the loss of beneficial microbial diversity [124, 125]. Research, by Kokalis-Burelle and his coworkers in the year 2006, shows that PGPR strains like *B. subtilis* GBO3 enhance fungal populations without harming native bacteria [126]. Sustainable agriculture is necessary for future food security. The **Figure 3**, highlights the bacterium abilities in maintenance of soil health.

6.2 Regulatory and safety considerations for agricultural and environmental uses

The development of novel biotechnology applications utilizing *B. subtilis* in a variety of sectors may encounter regulatory obstacles [127]. It might be difficult to scale up *B. subtilis* production for industrial uses without compromising quality. The variations in microbial behavior might make it challenging to get consistent yields

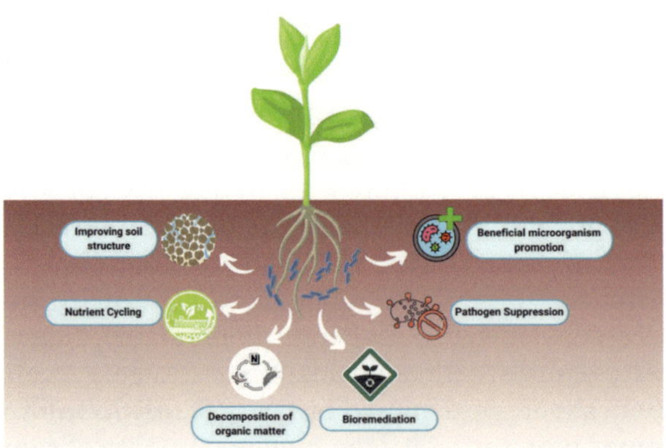

Figure 3.
Role of Bacillus subtilis *in soil health.*

of desired bioproducts. In a variety of environments, *B. subtilis* struggles with other microorganisms for resources and habitats [128]. The environmental stresses like as variations in pH, temperature, and nutrition availability must be tolerated by the microorganism [129]. The possibility exists that *B. subtilis* may acquire genes resistant to antibiotics, thereby causing harm to ecosystems [113].

7. Conclusion and future research directions

B. subtilis elevates plant growth and defense mechanisms and maintains sustainability in the environment through the production of a plethora of antimicrobial compounds [130–132]. There is an urgent need for whatever knowledge we have on *B. subtilis* to be integrated and explored in other domains of computer science, and engineering. The development of computer modeling, and systems biology can provide multidisciplinary approaches to comprehend the intricate relationships within this bacterium. These methods may be very helpful in developing bacterial strains with the appropriate characteristics, streamlining their production processes, and developing prediction models for the way the bacteria can be used in various environmental conditions as a PGPR or environmental remediator. Furthermore, the advances in CRISPR-Cas9 technology can provide an additional ability to modify the *B. subtilis* bacterium to optimize its capacities and boost its effectiveness in the synthesis of metabolites for more biotechnological applications.

Acknowledgements

The authors would like to thank MIT World Peace University.

Author contribution

All authors have contributed to the chapter.

Conflict of interest

There is no conflict of interest.

Author details

Sonam Shrirang Shinde, Viraj Vivek Gaonkar, Humaira Mushtaq Mukadam and Shikha Vikrant Gaikwad*
Department of Biosciences and Technology, School of Sciences and Environmental Studies, Faculty of Sciences and Health Sciences, Dr. Vishwanath Karad MIT World Peace University, Pune, Maharashtra, India

*Address all correspondence to: drshikhagaikwad@gmail.com

References

[1] Akinsemolu AA, Onyeaka H, Odion S, Adebanjo I. Exploring *Bacillus subtilis*: Ecology, biotechnological applications, and future prospects. Journal of Basic Microbiology. 2024;**64**(6):e202300614. DOI: 10.1002/jobm.202300614

[2] Errington J, Aart LT. Microbe profile: *Bacillus subtilis*: Model organism for cellular development, and industrial workhorse. Microbiology. 2020;**166**(5):425-427. DOI: 10.1099/mic.0.000922

[3] Gallegos-Monterrosa R, Christensen MN, Barchewitz T, Koppenhöfer S, Priyadarshini B, Bálint B, et al. Impact of rap-Phr system abundance on adaptation of *Bacillus subtilis*. Communications Biology. 2021;**4**(1):468. DOI: 10.1038/s42003-021-01983-9

[4] Qin Y, Angelini LL, Chai Y. *Bacillus subtilis* cell differentiation, biofilm formation and environmental prevalence. Microorganisms. 2022;**10**(6):1108. DOI: 10.3390/microorganisms10061108

[5] Stülke J, Grüppen A, Bramkamp M, Pelzer S. *Bacillus subtilis*, a swiss army knife in science and biotechnology. Journal of Bacteriology. 2023;**205**(5):e00102-e00123. DOI: 10.1128/jb.00102-23

[6] Shah V, Daverey A. Phytoremediation: A multidisciplinary approach to clean up heavy metal contaminated soil. Environmental Technology and Innovation. 2020;**18**:100774. DOI: 10.1016/j.eti.2020.100774

[7] Singh G, Pujari M. *Bacillus subtilis* as a plant-growth-promoting rhizobacteria: A review. Plant Archives (09725210). 2022;**22**(2):100-109. DOI: 10.51470/PLANTARCHIVES.2022.v22.no2.018

[8] Kejela T. Phytohormone-producing rhizobacteria and their role in plant growth. In: Basharat A, Javed I, editors. New Insights into Phytohormones. London, UK: IntechOpen; 2024. DOI: 10.5772/intechopen.1002823

[9] Chieb M, Gachomo EW. The role of plant growth promoting rhizobacteria in plant drought stress responses. BMC Plant Biology. 2023;**23**(1):407. DOI: 10.1186/s12870-023-04403-8

[10] Jiang L, Lee MH, Kim CY, Kim SW, Kim PI, Min SR, et al. Plant growth promotion by two volatile organic compounds emitted from the fungus *Cladosporium halotolerans* NGPF1. Frontiers in Plant Science. 2021;**12**:794349. DOI: 10.3389/fpls.2021.794349

[11] Tang J, Li Y, Zhang L, Mu J, Jiang Y, Fu H, et al. Biosynthetic pathways and functions of indole-3-acetic acid in microorganisms. Microorganisms. 2023;**11**(8):2077. DOI: 10.3390/microorganisms11082077

[12] Huang T, Zhang Y, Yu Z, Zhuang W, Zeng Z. Bacillus velezensis BV01 has broad-spectrum biocontrol potential and the ability to promote plant growth. Microorganisms. 2023;**11**(11):2627. DOI: 10.3390/microorganisms11112627

[13] Lim JH, Kim SD. Synergistic plant growth promotion by the indigenous auxins-producing PGPR *Bacillus subtilis* AH18 and *Bacillus licheniforims* K11. Journal of the Korean Society for Applied Biological Chemistry. 2009;**52**:531-538. DOI: 10.3839/jksabc.2009.090

[14] Duca DR, Glick BR. Indole-3-acetic acid biosynthesis and its regulation in plant-associated bacteria. Applied

Microbiology and Biotechnology. 2020;**104**:8607-8619. DOI: 10.1007/s00253-020-10869-5

[15] Wagi S, Ahmed A. *Bacillus spp.*: Potent microfactories of bacterial IAA. PeerJ. 2019;7:e7258. DOI: 10.7717/peerj.7258

[16] Chand K, Shah S, Pant B. Growth promoting effect of endophytic bacteria *Bacillus subtilis* from leaves of *Vanda cristata* and its potential impact on in vitro growth of orchid. Journal of Nepal Biotechnology Association. 2023;**4**(1):8-16. DOI: 10.3126/jnba.v4i1.53441

[17] Park S, Kim AL, Hong YK, Shin JH, Joo SH. A highly efficient auxin-producing bacterial strain and its effect on plant growth. Journal of Genetic Engineering and Biotechnology. 2021;**19**:1-9. DOI: 10.1186/s43141-021-00252-w

[18] Ji C, Wang X, Tian H, Hao L, Wang C, Zhou Y, et al. Effects of *bacillus methylotrophicus* M4-1 on physiological and biochemical traits of wheat under salinity stress. Journal of Applied Microbiology. 2020;**129**(3):695-711. DOI: 10.1111/jam.14644

[19] Minakshi SS, Sood G, Chauhan A. Optimization of IAA production and P-solubilization potential in *Bacillus subtilis* KA (1) 5r isolated from the medicinal herb *Aconitum heterophyllum*-growing in western Himalaya, India. Journal of Pharmacognosy and Phytochemistry. 2020;**9**(1):2008-2015

[20] Kotov AA, Kotova LM. Auxin/cytokinin antagonism in shoot development: From moss to seed plants. Journal of Experimental Botany. 2023;**74**(21):6391-6395. DOI: 10.1093/jxb/erad417

[21] Oleńska E, Małek W, Wójcik M, Swiecicka I, Thijs S, Vangronsveld J. Beneficial features of plant growth-promoting rhizobacteria for improving plant growth and health in challenging conditions: A methodical review. Science of the Total Environment. 2020;**743**:140682. DOI: 10.1016/j.scitotenv.2020.140682

[22] Mishra J, Singh R, Arora NK. Plant growth-promoting microbes: Diverse roles in agriculture and environmental sustainability. Probiotics and Plant Health. 2017;**1**:71-111. DOI: 10.1007/978-981-10-3473-2_4

[23] Orozco-Mosqueda MD, Santoyo G, Glick BR. Recent advances in the bacterial phytohormone modulation of plant growth. Plants. 2023;**12**(3):606. DOI: 10.3390/plants12030606

[24] Sorokan A, Veselova S, Benkovskaya G, Maksimov I. Endophytic strain *Bacillus subtilis* 26D increases levels of phytohormones and repairs growth of potato plants after Colorado potato beetle damage. Plants. 2021;**10**(5):923. DOI: 10.3390/plants10050923

[25] Kang SM, Hamayun M, Khan MA, Iqbal A, Lee IJ. *Bacillus subtilis* JW1 enhances plant growth and nutrient uptake of Chinese cabbage through gibberellins secretion. Journal of Applied Botany and Food Quality. 2019;**92**:172-178. DOI: 10.5073/JABFQ.2019.092.023

[26] Wang H, Wang S, He X, Xie M, Cai M, Zhu Y, et al. A promising product: Abscisic acid-producing bacterial agents for restricting cadmium enrichment in field vegetable crops. Food Chemistry: X. 2023;**19**:100795. DOI: 10.1016/j.fochx.2023.100795

[27] Nagrale DT, Chaurasia A, Kumar S, Gawande SP, Hiremani NS, Shankar R, et al. PGPR: The treasure of multifarious beneficial microorganisms for nutrient mobilization, pest biocontrol and plant growth promotion in field

crops. World Journal of Microbiology and Biotechnology. 2023;**39**(4):100. DOI: 10.1007/s11274-023-03536-0

[28] Stevens CJ. Nitrogen in the environment. Science. 2019;**363**(6427): 578-580. DOI: 10.1126/science.aav8215

[29] Korir H, Mungai NW, Thuita M, Hamba Y, Masso C. Co-inoculation effect of rhizobia and plant growth promoting rhizobacteria on common bean growth in a low phosphorus soil. Frontiers in Plant Science. 2017;**8**:141. DOI: 10.3389/fpls.2017.00141

[30] Sun B, Bai Z, Bao L, Xue L, Zhang S, Wei Y, et al. *Bacillus subtilis* biofertilizer mitigating agricultural ammonia emission and shifting soil nitrogen cycling microbiomes. Environment International. 2020;**144**:105989. DOI: 10.1016/j.envint.2020.105989

[31] Sun BO, Gu L, Bao L, Zhang S, Wei Y, Bai Z, et al. Application of biofertilizer containing *Bacillus subtilis* reduced the nitrogen loss in agricultural soil. Soil Biology and Biochemistry. 2020;**148**:107911. DOI: 10.1016/j.soilbio.2020.107911

[32] Khan F, Siddique AB, Shabala S, Zhou M, Zhao C. Phosphorus plays key roles in regulating plants' physiological responses to abiotic stresses. Plants. 2023;**12**(15):2861. DOI: 10.3390/plants12152861

[33] Alori ET, Glick BR, Babalola OO. Microbial phosphorus solubilization and its potential for use in sustainable agriculture. Frontiers in Microbiology. 2017;**8**:971. DOI: 10.3389/fmicb.2017.00971

[34] Jensen CN, Pang JK, Gottardi M, Kračun SK, Svendsen BA, Nielsen KF, et al. *Bacillus subtilis* promotes plant phosphorus (P) acquisition through P solubilization and stimulation of root and root hair growth. Physiologia Plantarum. 2024;**176**(3):e14338. DOI: 10.1111/ppl.14338

[35] Khatoon N, Khan M. Evaluation of *Bacillus subtilis* MRB4, as plant growth promoter and potential phosphate solubilizer under abiotic stress. Journal of Applied Biology and Biotechnology. 2020;**8**(5):27-35. DOI: 10.7324/JABB.2020.80504

[36] Emami S, Alikhani HA, Pourbabaee AA, Etesami H, MotasharezadehB,SarmadianF.Consortium of endophyte and rhizosphere phosphate solubilizing bacteria improves phosphorous use efficiency in wheat cultivars in phosphorus deficient soils. Rhizosphere. 2020;**14**:100196. DOI: 10.1016/j.rhisph.2020.100196

[37] Radhakrishnan R, Hashem A, Abd_Allah EF. Bacillus: A biological tool for crop improvement through bio-molecular changes in adverse environments. Frontiers in Physiology. 2017;**8**:667. DOI: 10.3389/fphys.2017.00667

[38] Ahmad M, Ahmad I, Hilger TH, Nadeem SM, Akhtar MF, Jamil M, et al. Preliminary study on phosphate solubilizing *Bacillus subtilis* strain Q3 and Paeni *Bacillus sp*. strain Q6 for improving cotton growth under alkaline conditions. PeerJ. 2018;**6**:e5122. DOI: 10.7717/peerj.5122

[39] Iqbal Z, Ahmad M, Raza MA, Hilger T, Rasche F. Phosphate-solubilizing bacillus sp. modulate soil exoenzyme activities and improve wheat growth. Microbial Ecology. 2024;**87**(1):31. DOI: 10.1007/s00248-023-02340-5

[40] Wang XQ, Zhao DL, Shen LL, Jing CL, Zhang CS. Application and

mechanisms of *Bacillus subtilis* in biological control of plant disease. In: Role of Rhizospheric Microbes in Soil: Volume 1: Stress Management and Agricultural Sustainability. 2018. pp. 225-250. DOI: 10.1007/978-981-10-8402-7_9

[41] Awan ZA, Shoaib A, Schenk PM, Ahmad A, Alansi S, Paray BA. Antifungal potential of volatiles produced by *Bacillus subtilis* BS-01 against *Alternaria solani* in *Solanum lycopersicum*. Frontiers in Plant Science. 2023;**13**:1089562. DOI: 10.3389/fpls.2022.1089562

[42] Jan F, Arshad H, Ahad M, Jamal A, Smith DL. In vitro assessment of *Bacillus subtilis* FJ3 affirms its biocontrol and plant growth promoting potential. Frontiers in Plant Science. 2023;**14**:1205894. DOI: 10.3389/fpls.2023.1205894

[43] Riaz R, Khan A, Khan WJ, Jabeen Z, Yasmin H, Naz R, et al. Vegetable associated *Bacillus spp*. suppress the pea (*Pisum sativum* L.) root rot caused by *Fusarium solani*. Biological Control. 2021;**158**:104610. DOI: 10.1016/j.biocontrol.2021.104610

[44] Rashad YM, Abdalla SA, Sleem MM. Endophytic *Bacillus subtilis* SR22 triggers defense responses in tomato against rhizoctonia root rot. Plants. 2022;**11**(15):2051. DOI: 10.3390/plants11152051

[45] Amin HA, El Kammar HF, Saied SM, Soliman AM. Effect of *Bacillus subtilis* on *potato virus Y* (PVY) disease resistance and growth promotion in potato plants. European Journal of Plant Pathology. 2023;**167**(4):743-758. DOI: 10.1007/s10658-023-02774-0

[46] Khedher SB, Mejdoub-Trabelsi B, Tounsi S. Biological potential of *Bacillus subtilis* V26 for the control of *Fusarium wilt* and tuber dry rot on potato caused by *Fusarium* species and the promotion of plant growth. Biological Control. 2021;**152**:104444. DOI: 10.1016/j.biocontrol.2020.104444

[47] Cozzolino ME, Distel JS, García PA, Mascotti ML, Ayub MJ, Benazzi LM, et al. Control of postharvest fungal pathogens in pome fruits by lipopeptides from a *Bacillus sp*. isolate SL-6. Scientia Horticulturae. 2020;**261**:108957. DOI: 10.1016/j.scienta.2019.108957

[48] Samaras A, Karaoglanidis GS, Tzelepis G. Insights into the multitrophic interactions between the biocontrol agent *Bacillus subtilis* MBI 600, the pathogen *Botrytis cinerea* and their plant host. Microbiological Research. 2021;**248**:126752. DOI: 10.1016/j.micres.2021.126752

[49] Zhang Q, Stummer BE, Guo Q, Zhang W, Zhang X, Zhang L, et al. Quantification of *pseudomonas protegens* FD6 and *Bacillus subtilis* NCD-2 in soil and the wheat rhizosphere and suppression of root pathogenic *Rhizoctonia solani* AG-8. Biological Control. 2021;**154**:104504. DOI: 10.1016/j.biocontrol.2020.104504

[50] Latha P, Karthikeyan M, Rajeswari E. Endophytic bacteria: Prospects and applications for the plant disease management. In: Plant Health under Biotic Stress: Volume 2: Microbial Interactions. 2019. pp. 1-50. DOI: 10.1007/978-981-13-6040-4_1

[51] Dimkić I, Janakiev T, Petrović M, Degrassi G, Fira D. Plant-associated bacillus and pseudomonas antimicrobial activities in plant disease suppression via biological control mechanisms-a review. Physiological and Molecular Plant Pathology. 2022;**117**:101754. DOI: 10.1016/j.pmpp.2021.101754

[52] Etesami H, Jeong BR, Glick BR. Biocontrol of plant diseases by *Bacillus*

spp. Physiological and Molecular Plant Pathology. 2023;**126**:102048. DOI: 10.1016/j.pmpp.2023.102048

[53] Andrić S, Meyer T, Ongena M. Bacillus responses to plant-associated fungal and bacterial communities. Frontiers in Microbiology. 2020;**11**:1350. DOI: 10.3389/fmicb.2020.01350

[54] Putri RE, Mubarik NR, Ambarsari L, Wahyudi AT. The disease suppression of soybean (var. Grobogan) by the implementation of *Bacillus subtilis* strain CR. 9 antifungal compounds nanoemulsion. Journal of the Saudi Society of Agricultural Sciences. 2023;**22**(6):384-393. DOI: 10.1016/j.jssas.2023.03.004

[55] Hoff G, Arguelles Arias A, Boubsi F, Pršić J, Meyer T, Ibrahim HM, et al. Surfactin stimulated by pectin molecular patterns and root exudates acts as a key driver of the Bacillus-plant mutualistic interaction. MBio. 2021;**12**(6):e01774-e01721. DOI: 10.1128/mBio.01774-21

[56] Lajis AF. Biomanufacturing process for the production of bacteriocins from Bacillaceae family. Bioresources and Bioprocessing. 2020;**7**:1-26. DOI: 10.1186/s40643-020-0295-z

[57] Muras A, Romero M, Mayer C, Otero A. Biotechnological applications of *Bacillus licheniformis*. Critical Reviews in Biotechnology. 2021;**41**(4):609-627. DOI: 10.1080/07388551.2021.1873239

[58] Blake C, Christensen MN, Kovács ÁT. Molecular aspects of plant growth promotion and protection by *Bacillus subtilis*. Molecular Plant-Microbe Interactions. 2021;**34**(1):15-25. DOI: 10.1094/MPMI-08-20-0225-CR

[59] Kenneth OC, Nwadibe EC, Kalu AU, Unah UV. Plant growth promoting rhizobacteria (PGPR): A novel agent for sustainable food production. American Journal of Agricultural and Biological Sciences. 2019;**14**(35):54. DOI: 10.3844/ajabssp.2019.35.54

[60] Brzezinska MS, Kalwasińska A, Świątczak J, Żero K, Jankiewicz U. Exploring the properties of chitinolytic Bacillus isolates for the pathogens biological control. Microbial Pathogenesis. 2020;**148**:104462. DOI: 10.1016/j.micpath.2020.104462

[61] Pandey C, Prabha D, Negi YK, Maheshwari DK, Dheeman S, Gupta M. Macrolactin A mediated biocontrol of *Fusarium oxysporum* and *Rhizoctonia solani* infestation on *Amaranthus hypochondriacus* by *Bacillus subtilis* BS-58. Frontiers in Microbiology. 2023;**14**:1105849. DOI: 10.3389/fmicb.2023.1105849

[62] Deb CR, Tatung M. Siderophore producing bacteria as biocontrol agent against phytopathogens for a better environment: A review. South African Journal of Botany. 2024;**165**:153-162. DOI: 10.1016/j.sajb.2023.12.031

[63] Ghazy N, El-Nahrawy S. Siderophore production by *Bacillus subtilis* MF497446 and *Pseudomonas koreensis* MG209738 and their efficacy in controlling *Cephalosporium maydis* in maize plant. Archives of Microbiology. 2021;**203**(3):1195-1209. DOI: 10.1007/s00203-020-02113-5

[64] Nithyapriya S, Lalitha S, Sayyed RZ, Reddy MS, Dailin DJ, El Enshasy HA, et al. Production, purification, and characterization of bacillibactin siderophore of *Bacillus subtilis* and its application for improvement in plant growth and oil content in sesame. Sustainability. 2021;**13**(10):5394. DOI: 10.3390/su13105394

[65] Chandwani S, Dewala S, Chavan SM, Paul D, Pachaiappan R, Gopi M, et al. Complete genome sequencing of *Bacillus subtilis* (CWTS 5), a siderophore-producing bacterium triggers antagonistic potential against *Ralstonia solanacearum*. Journal of Applied Microbiology. 2023;**134**(4):lxad066. DOI: 10.1093/jambio/lxad066

[66] Gowda AA, Pankaj SD, Singh AK, Sowmya R. Nematicidal potential of plant growth-promoting rhizobacteria against *Meloidogyne incognita* infesting tomato under protected cultivation. Egyptian Journal of Biological Pest Control. 2022;**32**(1):145. DOI: 10.1186/s41938-022-00643-2

[67] Samaniego-Gámez BY, Valle-Gough RE, Garruña-Hernández R, Reyes-Ramírez A, Latournerie-Moreno L, Tun-Suárez JM, et al. Induced systemic resistance in the *Bacillus spp*.—Capsicum chinense Jacq. —PepGMV interaction, elicited by defense-related gene expression. Plants. 2023;**12**(11):2069. DOI: 10.3390/plants12112069

[68] Rumyantsev SD, Veselova SV, Burkhanova GF, Alekseev VY, Maksimov IV. *Bacillus subtilis* 26D triggers induced systemic resistance against *Rhopalosiphum padi* L. by regulating the expression of genes AGO, DCL and microRNA in bread spring wheat. Microorganisms. 2023;**11**(12):2983. DOI: 10.3390/microorganisms11122983

[69] Jin Y, Zhu H, Luo S, Yang W, Zhang L, Li S, et al. Role of maize root exudates in promotion of colonization of *Bacillus velezensis* strain S3-1 in rhizosphere soil and root tissue. Current Microbiology. 2019;**76**:855-862. DOI: 10.1007/s00284-019-01699-4

[70] Sagar A, Yadav SS, Sayyed RZ, Sharma S, Ramteke PW. Bacillus subtilis: A multifarious plant growth promoter, biocontrol agent, and bioalleviator of abiotic stress. In: Bacilli in Agrobiotechnology: Plant Stress Tolerance, Bioremediation, and Bioprospecting. Cham: Springer International Publishing; 2022. pp. 561-580. DOI: 10.1007/978-3-030-85465-2_24

[71] Samaras A, Nikolaidis M, Antequera-GómezML,Cámara-AlmirónJ, Romero D, Moschakis T, et al. Whole genome sequencing and root colonization studies reveal novel insights in the biocontrol potential and growth promotion by *Bacillus subtilis* MBI 600 on cucumber. Frontiers in Microbiology. 2021;**11**:600393. DOI: 10.3389/fmicb.2020.600393

[72] Pertile M, Antunes JE, Araujo FF, Mendes LW, Van den Brink PJ, Araujo AS. Responses of soil microbial biomass and enzyme activity to herbicides imazethapyr and flumioxazin. Scientific Reports. 2020;**10**(1):7694. DOI: 10.1038/s41598-020-64648-3

[73] Pelosi C, Bertrand C, Daniele G, Coeurdassier M, Benoit P, Nélieu S, et al. Residues of currently used pesticides in soils and earthworms: A silent threat? Agriculture, Ecosystems and Environment. 2021;**305**:107167. DOI: 10.1016/j.agee.2020.107167

[74] Syromyatnikov MY, Isuwa MM, Savinkova OV, Derevshchikova MI, Popov VN. The effect of pesticides on the microbiome of animals. Agriculture. 2020;**10**(3):79. DOI: 10.3390/agriculture10030079

[75] Kumar J, Ramlal A, Mallick D, Mishra V. An overview of some biopesticides and their importance in plant protection for commercial acceptance. Plants. 2021;**10**(6):1185. DOI: 10.3390/plants10061185

[76] Abuhena M, Al-Rashid J, Azim MF, Khan MN, Kabir MG, Barman NC, et al. Optimization of industrial (3000 L) production of *Bacillus subtilis* CW-S and its novel application for minituber and industrial-grade potato cultivation. Scientific Reports. 2022;**12**(1):11153. DOI: 10.1038/s41598-022-15366-5

[77] Arthurs S, Dara SK. Microbial biopesticides for invertebrate pests and their markets in the United States. Journal of Invertebrate Pathology. 2019;**165**:13-21. DOI: 10.1016/j.jip.2018.01.008

[78] Nimrat S, Lookchan S, Boonthai T, Vuthiphandchai V. Bioremediation of petroleum contaminated soils by lipopeptide producing *Bacillus subtilis* SE1. African Journal of Biotechnology. 2019;**18**(23):494-501. DOI: 10.5897/AJB2019.16822

[79] Wróbel M, Śliwakowski W, Kowalczyk P, Kramkowski K, Dobrzyński J. Bioremediation of heavy metals by the genus *Bacillus*. International Journal of Environmental Research and Public Health. 2023;**20**(6):4964. DOI: 10.3390/ijerph20064964

[80] Mohsin MZ, Omer R, Huang J, Mohsin A, Guo M, Qian J, et al. Advances in engineered *Bacillus subtilis* biofilms and spores, and their applications in bioremediation, biocatalysis, and biomaterials. Synthetic and Systems Biotechnology. 2021;**6**(3):180-191. DOI: 10.1016/j.synbio.2021.07.002

[81] Ghosh S, Bhattacharya J, Nitnavare R, Webster TJ. Heavy metal removal by Bacillus for sustainable agriculture. In: Bacilli in Agrobiotechnology: Plant Stress Tolerance, Bioremediation, and Bioprospecting. Cham: Springer International Publishing; 2022. pp. 1-30. DOI: 10.1007/978-3-030-85465-2_1

[82] Kanamarlapudi SLRK, Chintalpudi VK, Muddada S. Application of Biosorption for Removal of Heavy Metals from Wastewater. London, UK: IntechOpen; 2018. DOI: 10.5772/intechopen.77315

[83] Ayangbenro AS, Babalola OO. A new strategy for heavy metal polluted environments: A review of microbial biosorbents. International Journal of Environmental Research and Public Health. 2017;**14**(1):94. DOI: 10.3390/ijerph14010094

[84] Ponia V, Kumar H, Ishtiyaq S, Goswami R, Bhadauria S. Remediation of cadmium ions from the contaminated aqueous media by using dead biomass of *Bacillus subtilis*. International Journal of Advanced Research. 2022;**10**:344-359. DOI: 10.21474/IJAR01/14715

[85] Zhu X, Xiang Q, Chen L, Chen J, Wang L, Jiang N, et al. Engineered *Bacillus subtilis* biofilm@biochar living materials for in-situ sensing and bioremediation of heavy metal ions pollution. Journal of Hazardous Materials. 2024;**465**:133119. DOI: 10.1016/j.jhazmat.2023.133119

[86] Mardiyono M, Hidayati N. Bioremediation of chrome heavy metals on metal coating waste with *Bacillus subtilis* bacteria. In: International Conference on Science and Applied Science (ICSAS2020), Surakarta, Indonesia. Vol. 2296. 2020. p. 020033. DOI: 10.1063/5.0030561

[87] Saez JM, Casillas García V, Polti MA, Benimeli CS. Microemulsions as a novel tool for enhancing the bioremediation of xenobiotics. Microbial Metabolism of Xenobiotic Compounds. 2019;**10**:305-317. DOI: 10.1007/978-981-13-7462-3_15

[88] Eras-Muñoz E, Farré A, Sánchez A, Font X, Gea T. Microbial biosurfactants:

A review of recent environmental applications. Bioengineered. 2022;**13**(5):12365-12391. DOI: 10.1080/21655979.2022.2074621

[89] Sansinenea E, Ortiz A. Secondary metabolites of soil *Bacillus spp*. Biotechnology Letters. 2011;**33**:1523-1538. DOI: 10.1007/s10529-011-0617-5

[90] Bekele GK, Gebrie SA, Mekonen E, Fida TT, Woldesemayat AA, Abda EM, et al. Isolation and characterization of diesel-degrading bacteria from hydrocarbon-contaminated sites, flower farms, and Soda Lakes. International Journal of Microbiology. 2022;**2022**(1):5655767. DOI: 10.1155/2022/5655767

[91] Pathogens, precipitation and produce prices. Nature Climate Change. 2021;**11**:635. DOI: 10.1038/s41558-021-01124-4

[92] Andryukov BG, Karpenko AA, Lyapun IN. Learning from nature: Bacterial spores as a target for current technologies in medicine (review). Sovremennye Tehnologii V Medicine. 2020;**12**:105. DOI: 10.17691/stm2020.12.3.13

[93] Tiwari S, Prasad V, Lata C. Bacillus: Plant growth promoting bacteria for sustainable agriculture and environment. In: Singh JS, Singh DP, editors. New and Future Developments in Microbial Biotechnology and Bioengineering. Elsevier; 2019. pp. 43-55. DOI: 10.1016/B978-0-444-64191-5.00003-1

[94] Khan AR, Mustafa A, Hyder S, Valipour M, Rizvi ZF, Gondal AS, et al. *Bacillus spp*. as bioagents: Uses and application for sustainable agriculture. Biology. 2022;**11**:1763. DOI: 10.3390/biology11121763

[95] Khan A, Singh AV, Gautam SS, Agarwal A, Punetha A, Upadhayay VK, et al. Microbial bioformulation: A microbial assisted biostimulating fertilization technique for sustainable agriculture. Frontiers in Plant Science. 2023;**14**:1270039. DOI: 10.3389/fpls.2023.1270039

[96] Kiruba N, Michellin J, Saeid A. An insight into microbial inoculants for bioconversion of waste biomass into sustainable "bio-organic" fertilizers: A bibliometric analysis and systematic literature review. International Journal of Molecular Sciences. 2022;**23**(21):13049. DOI: 10.3390/ijms232113049

[97] Chenikher S, Guez JS, Coutte F, Pekpe M, Jacques P, Cassar JP. Control of the specific growth rate of *Bacillus subtilis* for the production of biosurfactant lipopeptides in bioreactors with foam overflow. Process Biochemistry. 2010;**45**:1800-1807. DOI: 10.1016/j.procbio.2010.06.001

[98] Stamenkovic-Stojanovic S, Karabegović IT, Beškoski V, NikolićN, LazićM. Bacillusbasedmicrobial formulations: Optimization of the production process. Hemijska industrija. 2019;**73**:14-14. DOI: 10.2298/HEMIND190214014S

[99] Schisler DA, Slininger PJ, Behle RW, Jackson MA. Formulation of *Bacillus spp*. for biological control of plant diseases. Phytopathology. 2004;**94**:1267-1271. DOI: 10.1094/PHYTO.2004.94.11.1267

[100] El-Hassan SA, Gowen SR. Formulation and delivery of the bacterial antagonist *Bacillus subtilis* for management of lentil vascular wilt caused by *Fusarium oxysporum* f. sp. lentis. Journal of Phytopathology. 2006;**154**:148-155. DOI: 10.1111/j.1439-0434.2006.01075.x

[101] Paulitz T. Biological control of damping-off diseases with seed treatments. In: Tjamos ES, Papavizas GC, Cook RJ, editors. Biological Control of Plant Diseases: Progress and Challenges for the Future. New York, NY, USA: Plenum Press; 1992. pp. 145-156. DOI: 10.1007/978-1-4757-9468-7_20

[102] Roberti R, Selmi C. Biological control of plant pathogens by *Bacillus subtilis*. Informatore Fitopatologico. 1999;**49**:15-21. DOI: 10.5555/20001002785

[103] Amein T, SAI W, Wikström M, Koch E, Schmitt A, Stephan D, et al. Evaluation of non-chemical seed treatment methods for control of *Alternaria brassicicola* on cabbage seeds. Journal of Plant Diseases and Protection. 2011;**118**:214-221. DOI: 10.1007/BF03356406

[104] Mancini V, Romanazzi G. Seed treatments to control seedborne fungal pathogens of vegetable crops. Pest Management Science. 2013;**70**:860-868. DOI: 10.1002/ps.3693

[105] Mousavi M, Omidi H. Seed priming with bio-priming improves stand establishment, seed germination and salinity tolerance in canola cultivar (Hayola 401). Iranian Journal of Plant Physiology. 1 May 2019;**9**(3):2807-2817. DOI: magiran.com/p2019705

[106] El-Gendi H, Al-Askar AA, Király L, Samy MA, Moawad H, Abdelkhalek A. Foliar applications of *Bacillus subtilis* HA1 culture filtrate enhance tomato growth and induce systemic resistance against *tobacco mosaic virus* infection. Horticulturae. 2022;**8**:301. DOI: 10.3390/horticulturae8040301

[107] Kordatzaki G, Katsenios N, Giannoglou M, Andreou V, Chanioti S, Katsaros G, et al. Effect of foliar and soil application of plant growth promoting bacteria on kale production and quality characteristics. Scientia Horticulturae. 2022;**301**:111094. DOI: 10.1016/j.scienta.2022.111094

[108] Santivarangkna C, Kulozik U, Foerst P. Alternative drying processes for the industrial preservation of lactic acid starter cultures. Biotechnology Progress. 2007;**23**(2):302-315. DOI: 10.1021/bp060268f

[109] Abadias M, Teixidó N, Usall J, Solsona C, Viñas I. Survival of the postharvest biocontrol yeast *Candida sake* CPA-1 after dehydration by spray-drying. Biocontrol Science and Technology. 2005;**15**(8):835-846. DOI: 10.1080/09583150500187041

[110] Yánez-Mendizábal V, Viñas I, Usall J, Torres R, Solsona C, Abadias M, et al. Formulation development of the biocontrol agent *Bacillus subtilis* strain CPA-8 by spray-drying. Journal of Applied Microbiology. 2012;**112**(5):954-965. DOI: 10.1111/j.1365-2672.2012.05258.x

[111] Ahmed T, Noman M, Rizwan M, Ali S, Ijaz U, Nazir MM, et al. Green molybdenum nanoparticles-mediated bio-stimulation of *Bacillus sp*. strain ZH16 improved the wheat growth by managing in planta nutrients supply, ionic homeostasis and arsenic accumulation. Journal of Hazardous Materials. 2022;**423**:127024. DOI: 10.1016/j.jhazmat.2021.127024

[112] Kalam S, Basu A, Podile AR. Functional and molecular characterization of plant growth promoting Bacillus isolates from tomato rhizosphere. Heliyon. 2020;**6**:e04734. DOI: 10.1016/j.heliyon.2020.e04734

[113] Mahapatra S, Yadav R, Ramakrishna W. *Bacillus subtilis* impact

on plant growth, soil health and environment: Dr. Jekyll and Mr. Hyde. Journal of Applied Microbiology. 2022;**132**:3543-3562. DOI: 10.1111/jam.15480

[114] Ng CW, Yan WH, Tsim KW, San So P, Xia YT, To CT. Effects of *Bacillus subtilis* and *Pseudomonas fluorescens* as the soil amendment. Heliyon. 2022;**8**(11):e11674. DOI: 10.1016/j.heliyon.2022.e11674

[115] Su Y, Liu C, Fang H, et al. *Bacillus subtilis*: A universal cell factory for industry, agriculture, biomaterials and medicine. Microbial Cell Factories. 2020;**19**:173. DOI: 10.1186/s12934-020-01436-8

[116] Gu Y, Xu X, Wu Y, Niu T, Liu Y, Li J, et al. Advances and prospects of *Bacillus subtilis* cellular factories: From rational design to industrial applications. Metabolic Engineering. 2018;**50**:109-121. DOI: 10.1016/j.ymben.2018.05.006

[117] Soumare A, Boubekri K, Lyamlouli K, Hafidi M, Ouhdouch Y, Kouisni L. From isolation of phosphate solubilizing microbes to their formulation and use as biofertilizers: Status and needs. Frontiers in Bioengineering and Biotechnology. 2020;**7**:425. DOI: 10.3389/fbioe.2019.00425

[118] Schmidt JE, Gaudin AC. What is the agronomic potential of biofertilizers for maize? A meta-analysis. FEMS Microbiology Ecology. 2018;**94**(7):fiy094. DOI: 10.1093/femsec/fiy094

[119] Suganya V, Anuradha V. Microencapsulation and nanoencapsulation: A review. International Journal of Pharmaceutical and Clinical Research. 2017;**9**(3):233-239. DOI: 10.25258/ijpcr.v9i3.8324

[120] Feng C, Lü S, Gao C, Wang X, Xu X, Bai X, et al. “Smart” fertilizer with temperature-and pH-responsive behavior via surface-initiated polymerization for controlled release of nutrients. ACS Sustainable Chemistry and Engineering. 2015;**3**(12):3157-3166. DOI: 10.1021/acssuschemeng.5b01384

[121] Bejarano A, Puopolo G. Bioformulation of microbial biocontrol agents for a sustainable agriculture. In: Cal AD, Melgarejo P, Magan N, editors. How Research Can Stimulate the Development of Commercial Biological Control against Plant Diseases. Progress in Biological Control. Vol. 21. Cham: Springer; 2020. DOI: 10.1007/978-3-030-53238-3_16

[122] Silva MGC, Medeiros AO, Converti A, Almeida FCG, Sarubbo LA. Biosurfactants: Promising biomolecules for agricultural applications. Sustainability. 2024;**16**(1):449. DOI: 10.3390/su16010449

[123] Vishnu M, Malaisamy K, Soundararajan RP, Suganthi A, Subramanian A, Senthilkumar M, et al. Nano-bioformulations: Emerging trends and potential applications in next generation crop protection. Environmental Science: Nano. 2024;**11**:2831-2860. DOI: 10.1039/d4en00263f

[124] Behl K, Jaiswal P, Pabbi S. Recent advances in microbial and nano-formulations for effective delivery and agriculture sustainability. Biocatalysis and Agricultural Biotechnology. 2024;**58**:103180. DOI: 10.1016/j.bcab.2024.103180

[125] Khatoon Z, Huang S, Rafique M, Fakhar A, Kamran MA, Santoyo G. Unlocking the potential of plant growth-promoting rhizobacteria on soil health and the sustainability of agricultural

systems. Journal of Environmental Management. 2020;**273**:111118. DOI: 10.1016/j.jenvman.2020.111118

[126] Kokalis-Burelle N, Kloepper JW, Reddy MS. Plant growth-promoting rhizobacteria as transplant amendments and their effects on indigenous rhizosphere microorganisms. Applied Soil Ecology. 2006;**31**(1-2):91-100. DOI: 10.1016/j.apsoil.2005.03.007

[127] Elshaghabee FMF, Rokana N, Gulhane RD, Sharma C, Panwar H. *Bacillus* as potential probiotics: Status, concerns, and future perspectives. Frontiers in Microbiology. 2017;**8**:1490. DOI: 10.3389/fmicb.2017.01490

[128] Gonzalez-Covarrubias V, Martínez-Martínez E, del Bosque-Plata L. The potential of metabolomics in biomedical applications. Metabolites. 2022;**12**(2):194. DOI: 10.3390/metabo12020194

[129] Etesami H, Jeong BR, Glick BR. Potential use of *Bacillus spp*. as an effective biostimulant against abiotic stresses in crops—A review. Current Research in Biotechnology. 2023;**5**:100128. DOI: 10.1016/j.crbiot.2023.100128

[130] Wu Y, Guo W, Zhao J, Ding L, Chen X. Isolation and identification of a novel LCI like antibacterial protein from *Bacillus sp*. MD-5 reveals its potential application in controlling Staphylococcus aureus in food industry. Food Control. 2018;**89**:142-149. DOI: 10.1016/j.foodcont.2018.01.026

[131] Sevim A, Kutalmış A, Yabaneri C. Isolation, Molecular Characterization, and Antimicrobial Activity of the Members of the Family Bacillaceae Obtained from Soil Samples: Antimicrobial Activity of the Members of the Family Bacillaceae. 2022. DOI:10.36547/be.443

[132] Beneduzi A, Ambrosini A, Passaglia LM. Plant growth-promoting rhizobacteria (PGPR): Their potential as antagonists and biocontrol agents. Genetics and Molecular Biology. 2012;**35**:1044-1051. DOI: 10.1590/s1415-47572012000600020